CYSTIC FIBROSIS

A Guide for
Patient and Family

CYSTIC FIBROSIS

A Guide for
Patient and Family

David M. Orenstein, M.D.
Associate Professor of Pediatrics
University of Pittsburgh School of Medicine
and
Director, Cystic Fibrosis Center
Children's Hospital of Pittsburgh
Pittsburgh, Pennsylvania

Raven Press 🖎 **New York**

Raven Press, 1185 Avenue of the Americas, New York, New York 10036

Made in the United States of America

Library of Congress Cataloging-in-Publication Data

Orenstein, David M., 1945–
  Cystic fibrosis.

  Includes bibliography and index.
  1. Cystic fibrosis—Popular works.   I. Title.
[DNLM: 1. Cystic Fibrosis. WI 820 066c]
RC858.C95074   1989   616.3'7   86-42749
ISBN 0-88167-486-9 (soft)

The material contained in this volume was submitted as previously unpublished material, except in the instances in which some of the illustrative material was derived.

Great care has been taken to maintain the accuracy of the information contained in the volume. However, neither Raven Press nor the author can be held responsible for errors or for any consequences arising from the use of the information contained herein.

Cover design by Sam Patoine.

Quotation on opposite page taken, with permission, from the song, "What You Do With What You've Got," music and lyrics by Si Kahn, © Joe Hill Music, 1985.

*To all those patients and families who have so enriched my life,
and have taught me so well,*
    *"it's not just what you're given,
    but what you do with what you've got."*
                            Si Kahn

Preface

This book is written for all who have an interest in cystic fibrosis, whether they be patients, the friends and family of patients, or health professionals who work with patients and their families. It is designed to be of particular use to parents in the initial months that follow their child's diagnosis of cystic fibrosis. It is also written with the intention that it serve as a "refresher" course for people to review areas of treatment and physiology which they may have forgotten. The relatives and friends of a patient may also benefit from this introduction to cystic fibrosis.

An important group for whom this book is written is teenagers who were diagnosed in infancy. While teenagers grow up knowing a lot about cystic fibrosis, they seldom receive the in-depth explanation that their parents received immediately upon diagnosis. It is the author's hope that teenagers will use this book to gain more knowledge of cystic fibrosis. A final goal of this volume is to provide a foundation for understanding cystic fibrosis that will enable patients and families to understand more fully the advances that are rapidly being made in this field.

It is stressed throughout this book that cystic fibrosis is a serious disease, yet it is one that can be effectively controlled for long periods of time in most patients. It is a life-shortening disease, yet it is also one in which the outlook for patients' length and quality of life has improved dramatically in a relatively short time and continues to do so. It is a disease for which there is currently no cure, yet it is one for which treatment is very effective. It is a disease that creates demands on patients and families for daily treatments; it is also one in which the efforts of patients and families can greatly influence the health and quality of life of the patient. It is a disease that is commonly accepted as inhibiting normal life, yet the reality is that most patients go to school, play sports, and grow up accomplishing all the tasks, and experience all the joys and sorrows of childhood, adolescence, and young adulthood. It is the author's hope that patients and their families will find this volume to be of help in all these stages of life.

David Orenstein, M.D.

Acknowledgments

I want to offer thanks to a number of people who made this book possible:

My parents, Jacob and Florence Orenstein, who by their gentle example and instruction gave me an appreciation of the privilege of knowing and working with people;

My teachers, colleagues, and friends, Drs. Carl Doershuk, Bob Stern, Tom Boat, Bob Wood, and the late LeRoy Matthews, who by their example and instruction gave me an appreciation of the rewards of knowing and working with patients and families with cystic fibrosis;

My partner, Dr. Ed Pattishall, who gave many helpful suggestions for improving the manuscript;

My administrative assistant, Donna Wilding, who kept calm as we raced towards various deadlines;

My research partner and nurse, Dr. Pat Nixon and Liz Ross, who kept our research going despite my preoccupation with this book;

Louise Bauer and Doris Kanavos, Denise Rodgers, Gina Bucci, Julie Ryan, Peggy Gloninger, Mary Jane Slesinki, Karen Rezac, Dr. Geoff Kurland, and Dr. Joel Weinberg who make our own CF Center such a rewarding place in which to work;

Kathy Muffie, for her excellent illustrations;

The Caton, Johnston, and Michel families for taking the time and energy to read early versions of the manuscript;

And especially my wife, Susan Orenstein, M.D., for just about everything.

Contents

Contributors

Robert J. Beall, Ph.D. *Executive Vice President for Medical Affairs, Cystic Fibrosis Foundation, 931 Arlington Road, Bethesda, Maryland 20814*

Margaret F. Gloninger, M.S., R.D. *Assistant Professor of Nutrition, Department of Epidemiology, School of Public Health, University of Pittsburgh, Pittsburgh, Pennsylvania 15213*

Sherry Keramidas, Ph.D. *Associate Medical Director, Cystic Fibrosis Foundation, 931 Arlington Road, Bethesda, Maryland 20814*

David M. Orenstein, M.D. *Associate Professor of Pediatrics, Department of Pediatrics, University of Pittsburgh School of Medicine,* and *Director, Cystic Fibrosis Center and Pediatric Pulmonology Division, Children's Hospital of Pittsburgh, One Children's Place, 3705 Fifth Avenue at DeSoto Street, Pittsburgh, Pennsylvania 15213-3417*

Susan R. Orenstein, M.D. *Assistant Professor of Pediatrics, Division of Gastroenterology, Department of Pediatrics, University of Pittsburgh School of Medicine,* and *Cystic Fibrosis Center, Children's Hospital of Pittsburgh, One Children's Place, 3705 Fifth Avenue at DeSoto Street, Pittsburgh, Pennsylvania 15213-3417*

Denise R. Rodgers, M.S. *Instructor, Child Development, Community College of Allegheny County,* and *Child Development Specialist, Cystic Fibrosis Center, Children's Hospital of Pittsburgh, One Children's Place, 3705 Fifth Avenue at DeSoto Street, Pittsburgh, Pennsylvania 15213-3417*

Jean Homrighausen Zander, R.N., M.S.N. *Nurse Specialist, Pediatric/Pulmonary Section, Room 293, Riley Children's Hospital, 702 Barnhill Drive, Indianapolis, Indiana 46223*

CYSTIC FIBROSIS

A Guide for
Patient and Family

Introduction

David M. Orenstein

WHAT IS CYSTIC FIBROSIS?

Cystic fibrosis (CF) is a life-shortening, inherited disorder which affects the mucus-secreting glands of the body, especially affecting the mucus in the bronchial tubes of the lungs and in the small ducts of the pancreas. The lung problem can lead to progressive blockage, infection and lung damage, and even death if there is too much damage, while the pancreatic blockage causes poor digestion and poor absorption of food, leading to poor growth and undernutrition. The sweat glands are also affected, in that they secrete a much saltier sweat than normal. Anyone reading this book has probably heard about the sweat test used to diagnose CF. Mucus elsewhere is also affected, including in the reproductive tract in men and women with CF.

ARE ANY PARTS OF THE BODY NOT AFFECTED BY CF?

The list of body parts affected by CF can seem overwhelmingly long. But CF does *not* affect the brain and nervous system (it does *not* cause mental retardation); it does not affect the kidneys; it does not directly affect the heart; it does not affect the muscles; it does not affect the blood; and, except in the lungs, it does not interfere with the body's ability to fight infection.

WHAT CAUSES CYSTIC FIBROSIS?

Cystic fibrosis is an inherited disorder which is present from birth, although signs and symptoms of it may not show up for weeks, months, or even years after birth. Although it is inherited, the parents of a child with CF do not have CF, and most often there is no history of it in the family. Two CF genes are needed to cause CF, and it is inherited by receiving one CF gene from each parent. Each parent usually has only one CF gene, and thus has no sign of CF at all. Cystic fibrosis is very common among white

1

people, and is *the* most commonly inherited life-shortening disease, affecting 1 in every 2000 live babies born. One in 20 people carry the CF gene. CF is *not* caused by anything the parents did—or did not not do—during the pregnancy. *The only way to get CF is to inherit one CF gene from each parent.* You cannot "catch" CF; it is not contagious.

HOW LONG DO PEOPLE WITH CYSTIC FIBROSIS LIVE?

It is impossible to predict how long a patient will live. It *is* possible to give some overall statistics. Just a few decades ago, nearly all children with CF died before they reached 2 years of age. By 1986 (the latest year for which the information is available), the average survival had improved to age 26.5 years, with many people surviving into their 30's and 40's.

There are several important factors that explain the tremendous improvement, and that explain why the outlook continues to improve almost year by year. First, CF is a newly recognized disease. (It is not a *new* disease, as is related in Appendix D, but a newly *recognized* disease.) It was not until 1938 that Dr. Dorothy Andersen wrote the first medical paper describing a number of children who had died with digestive problems and lung problems. She was the first to recognize that this was not just a coincidence, but represented a single disease, which she called "cystic fibrosis of the pancreas." The name has been shortened to cystic fibrosis, but her description helped to lay the foundation for recognizing the disease, and therefore treating children who had it. Around this time, antibiotics were becoming available, and lung infections could be treated to a degree. In 1964, Drs. Doershuk and Matthews and their colleagues from Cleveland reported the results of 5 years of a comprehensive treatment program. These results were very much improved over previous results, and most modern treatment programs use the same basic principles which these pioneers used.

In the last 20 years, many new antibiotics have become available, making treatment more effective. Further, knowledge of CF has spread widely, so that now most pediatricians and family doctors are able to recognize the signs and symptoms of CF and are able to give children treatment while it can still be helpful, that is, before there is too much irreversible lung damage.

The point here is that the medical world has had good comprehensive treatment programs for patients with CF for only a little more than 20 years. This means that there are virtually no patients with CF who are 30 years old *and* were started on a treatment program in the first year of life. There are more and more teenagers and people in their 20's who were started on treatment programs early in life, before their lungs were in bad shape, and many of these young adults are doing extremely well. Therefore, there is every reason to be very optimistic about the future of a youngster diagnosed and started on treatment today. Certainly, while an average survival to age 26½ years reflects a tremendous improvement, it is not something to be satisfied with; but this is a situation which is continually improving.

RESEARCH AND THE BASIC DEFECT

At the time of the publication of this book, the basic defect in CF is not known. Much is understood about the kind of problems people have with CF, how to prevent many of those problems, and how to treat the problems that can't be prevented. But at a very basic chemical level, no one knows what exactly goes wrong within the cells of the body to cause the problems that occur. What this means for treatment is that the medications and therapies are all directed at *secondary* problems (problems that are themselves caused by the basic defect) and not at the underlying problem itself. Another way of putting it is that there is no *cure* for CF now, and almost certainly won't be until the basic biochemical/molecular problem is explained.

The situation is similar to that of diabetes. It is known that people get sick with diabetes because they don't have enough insulin to control their blood sugar. These people can lead normal lives by taking daily insulin shots, but they still have diabetes and will have it until scientists discover and eliminate the cause of inadequate insulin production.

Tremendous progress has been made in the search for the basic defect in CF. This is a very exciting time in CF research, because nearly every month an important piece of the puzzle is discovered and researchers get closer to identifying the cause of CF (current research issues are discussed in Chapter 12).

HOW CAN PEOPLE LEARN ABOUT CYSTIC FIBROSIS?

The purpose of this book is to provide information about all aspects of CF, including how it is inherited, the problems it causes, how it is treated, and current research. Cystic fibrosis centers and the Cystic Fibrosis Foundation can provide information also. Encyclopedias and many general medical books are *not* a good source of information, since they are likely to be out of date. Newspapers, especially the tabloids we all see in the checkout line in the grocery store, are also not good sources, for they are likely to announce the discovery of a cure that bears little relation to medical truth. Even if you hear something which sounds encouraging on a national TV news show, be sure to check it out with your CF center, or someone who is knowledgeable and up to date on research developments. There have been several instances of incorrect information—even dangerous information— being reported as medical truth on supposedly reputable news shows. In one of these instances, it was announced that CF was caused by a deficiency of selenium in the diet, and that a cure existed in taking huge doses of selenium; several babies died as a result of that report, after being given massive over-doses of selenium. Usually, information about CF that appears in the news is not harmful, and is even fairly accurate. But it is wise to be cautious about "dramatic breakthroughs" which are announced. Most often, medical progress is not made by dramatic breakthroughs but rather by tiny steps, with one group of scientists building upon the work of previous researchers. Your CF center and the CF Foundation are informed of all the reputable work in the field worldwide, and will be happy to provide you with this information.

ORGANIZATION OF THE BOOK

The goal of this book is to cover all the important topics that concern people with CF and their families. The opening chapter discusses the respiratory system (lungs), how it normally works, the changes brought about by CF, and the treatment of the lung problems. Chapter 2, on the digestive and gastrointestinal system, also reviews both normal functioning and that affected by cystic fibrosis. After these sections, there is a brief chapter on the other body systems affected by cystic fibrosis. Then follows a chapter on nutrition.

Chapter 5 discusses hospitalization and other types of elaborate treatments, and is followed by a short chapter dealing with various aspects of daily life including daycare, school, sports, home responsibilities, and travel. Exercise is considered separately in the following chapter. Next is a chapter on the genetics of CF, which describes the manner in which it is inherited, and then a chapter that deals with emotional and psychological issues (growing up with CF, effects on the family of a child with CF, etc.). The special problems of the adult with cystic fibrosis are discussed in Chapter 10. The next chapter discusses the difficult issues surrounding dying with CF.

Research—past, present, and future—is the subject of the next chapter. The national Cystic Fibrosis Foundation is discussed in Chapter 13.

The volume includes several appendices: a glossary of technical terms; a listing of commonly used medications, giving brand names and generic names, uses, and side effects; diagrams illustrating the proper techniques for performing chest physical therapy; a brief appendix on major historic landmarks in CF; a list of CF Centers in the United States; and a list of CF organizations worldwide.

The Respiratory System

David M. Orenstein

The respiratory system is the most important organ system for patients with cystic fibrosis (CF). Problems with this system account for over 95 percent of the sickness from CF, and also for more than 95 percent of the deaths from this disease. In the 50 years since CF was first recognized, treatment of lung disease has improved considerably, resulting in the tremendous improvement in longevity and quality of life that CF patients can now expect.

The three sections of this chapter are devoted to (1) a discussion of the normal anatomy and functioning of the respiratory system, (2) an explanation of how CF changes the functioning of this system, and (3) a review of the treatments that are aimed at preventing, correcting, or minimizing the changes that CF brings about in the respiratory system.

ANATOMY AND FUNCTION OF THE RESPIRATORY SYSTEM

All tissues in the body, especially the brain and exercising muscles, need oxygen to function. It is the task of the respiratory system to bring in oxygen from the air that surrounds us and transfer it to the bloodstream. Once in the bloodstream, the cardiovascular system (heart and blood vessels) delivers oxygen to all the parts of the body that need it. It is a further responsibility of the lungs to dispose of excess carbon dioxide which builds up in the process of normal metabolism. These tasks are essential to life, since all body tissues need oxygen to survive, and if too much carbon dioxide builds up in the bloodstream and brain, it can put someone so deeply to sleep that he or she will not breathe.

The Airways

The actual transfer of oxygen from the air we breathe to the bloodstream (and carbon dioxide from the blood to the air we exhale) takes place deep in

5

the lungs, in the **alveoli** (air sacs), which are located at the end of a long series of tubes. At the beginning of these air-carrying tubes, or "airways," are the nose and mouth, followed by the throat, then the larynx (or "voice-box," another name given to this area which includes the vocal cords), and the trachea (also called the "windpipe"). As the trachea enters the chest, it divides into two branches, and each branch leads into a lung. These branches are referred to as the **bronchial tubes**, or simply, **bronchi** (Fig. 1.1). Each bronchus reaches into its lung where it divides again, and yet again, forming a network of bronchi that extend into the various **lobes**, or sections, of the lung, and the *segments* of each lobe, the **subsegments** of each segment, etc. Each time the bronchi branch, they become smaller, and are thus able to distribute air to the smallest and farthest reaches of the lungs. [The word "branch" is frequently used to describe the bronchial system, for it does look very tree-like. Pulmonary physicians (lung specialists) and anatomists often adapt words used in forestry to describe this bronchial "tree."]

The bronchi divide, or branch, approximately 20 times before they reach the alveoli. It is in these air sacs that oxygen finally leaves the inhaled air and enters the bloodstream. Throughout most of this branching network, the bronchial tubes are referred to as "bronchi," or, for the smaller ones, "small bronchi." Toward the end of this network, however, the bronchi become

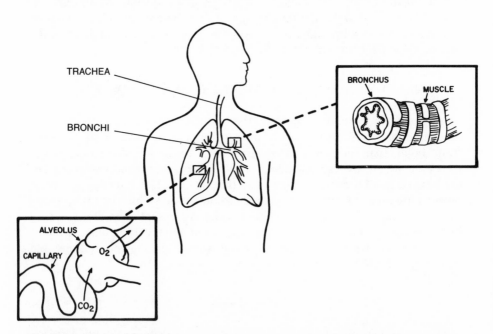

FIG. 1.1. The lungs, including bronchi and alveoli. Note the muscles in the bronchial wall. Oxygen enters the bloodstream by passing from the inhaled air through the wall of the alveoli and into the blood cells in the capillaries.

quite small and are referred to as **bronchioles**. Bronchioles are the last segment of tubes through which air passes before it reaches the alveoli.

The difference between bronchi and bronchioles, aside from their size, is that bronchi have **cartilage** in their walls and bronchioles don't. Both bronchi and bronchioles need something to stiffen their walls so that they maintain their shape and, particularly, so that they stay open. In healthy lungs, there is a tendency for the bronchi and bronchioles to enlarge slightly as the chest expands with each breath *inhaled,* and to narrow with each breath *exhaled.* If breathing is particularly strenuous, or if the support of the bronchial walls is not very strong, the bronchi and bronchioles can collapse during exhalation, making it difficult for the proper amount of air to leave the lungs.

In addition to cartilage, other tissues help support the bronchi. One of the most important is **muscle**: the bronchi and bronchioles have bands of muscle running around their walls. If a dangerous substance threatens to enter the lungs (such as a chemical with toxic fumes), these muscles can contract, squeezing down and making the bronchial opening much smaller than normal. With the bronchial passage blocked in this way, it is difficult for anything to get deeply into the bronchial tree. This action protects the lungs only if it happens briefly, and only if it happens when there is a true danger. However, this "protective" mechanism can actually be harmful if the bronchial muscles squeeze down at inappropriate times.

Gas Transfer and Delivery

The transfer of oxygen from the inhaled air to the bloodstream takes place at the alveoli. Running past each alveolus is a tiny blood vessel called a **pulmonary capillary**. The walls of the alveoli and the capillaries are membranes, so thin that oxygen and carbon dioxide can pass directly through them. It is through these walls that oxygen passes from the alveoli to the bloodstream, and that carbon dioxide passes from the bloodstream to the alveoli. There are 20 million of these tiny air sacs in a newborn infant's lungs, and 300 million in an adult. The enormity of these figures can be better grasped by imagining that, if you were to lay out the working surfaces between the alveoli and capillaries side-by-side, they would span an area the size of a tennis court.

After the oxygen has been supplied to the blood, the task remains of getting the blood to the tissues that need the oxygen (the brain, exercising muscles, etc.). Fortunately, there is an excellent system that accomplishes the task of pumping the blood to where it is needed. The pump, of course, is the heart.

Actually, the heart is a muscular double pump. The right side of the heart pumps blood through the lungs, where the blood becomes oxygenated through the process just described (and where the carbon dioxide is dumped out of the blood). After the **hemoglobin** molecules, which are the oxygen-carrying elements in the blood, are loaded with as much oxygen as possible (that is, they are fully *saturated* with oxygen), the blood flows back to the heart. It then enters the left side of the heart, where it is pumped to the rest of the body. Oxygen is removed from the blood by the tissues that need it. The deoxygenated blood then returns to the heart through the veins, and enters the right side of the heart. The heart then pumps the blood back to the lungs, where it is loaded with oxygen once again. At rest, an adult's heart will pump 4 to 5 liters of blood per minute (1 liter is approximately equal to a quart). During heavy exercise, that amount can increase to 25 or even to 30 liters per minute.

The condition can arise in which the oxygen levels are too low and the carbon dioxide levels are too high. This is called **respiratory failure**, and can result from several circumstances. If someone with normal lungs is paralyzed in a car accident, for example, the breathing muscles (see below, *The Respiratory Muscles*) could also become paralyzed and thus be unable to accomplish the work of breathing. Brain injury or brain disease, or drug overdoses, may also result in respiratory failure by damaging the brain's ability to direct the muscles to move the chest, in which case breathing will not occur. Serious lung disease can also cause respiratory failure if oxygen cannot be brought into, or carbon dioxide removed from, the bloodstream.

Control of Breathing

Among the many amazing things our body can do without our awareness is regulating how much we breathe. The main job of the lungs is to bring in the right amount of oxygen and eliminate the right amount of carbon dioxide that has been produced. This is a balancing act that is controlled with astounding precision.

In general, the more we breathe, the more oxygen we bring into the body, and the more carbon dioxide we breathe out. When we exercise, our muscles use as much as 10 to 20 times as much oxygen as when we're resting, and even more carbon dioxide is formed which needs to be eliminated. During strenuous exercise, we breathe 5 to 10 times as much air as when we're resting, and our heart pumps 5 or 6 times as much blood each minute, yet all the while the level of oxygen and carbon dioxide in the bloodstream remains almost exactly the same! You'd think that a little extra oxygen would come in, or not quite enough, or that a bit too much carbon dioxide would be breathed out, or not quite enough, but this doesn't happen. In healthy people as well as in most people with lung disease (including those with CF), the blood levels of oxygen and carbon dioxide are kept steady, regardless of what the person is doing.

This tight control is achieved by the brain's response to the two gases that the lungs manage—oxygen and carbon dioxide. Carbon dioxide is usually the more important regulator. If the breathing slows down (as it does in all of us now and then), less carbon dioxide will be breathed out and it will begin to build up in the body. As soon as this happens, the brain senses the buildup and sends the signal to the breathing muscles to breathe more, until the carbon dioxide level is back down to normal. The opposite occurs also: if the carbon dioxide level gets too low, the brain sends out the signal to slow down the breathing. Most of the time this is very fine tuning, requiring such small changes in breathing effort that we are usually unaware of the adjustments that are being made.

If the lungs are severely affected by disease and are not able to eliminate carbon dioxide effectively, the carbon dioxide level will build up and the brain will "instruct" the body to increase the rate and depth of breathing. After a period of time, however, the brain acts as though it has "gotten tired" of the message that the carbon dioxide level is too high, and it ignores the message. In its place, the brain will respond to another signal that regulates breathing—the oxygen level. It notices that the oxygen level is too low, and continues sending the message to the breathing muscles to increase breathing more. It is in this way that severe lung disease (from whatever cause) may alter the way the brain controls breathing patterns. Various drugs may also affect breathing patterns, either by making us breathe more, or by making us less sensitive to breathing commands, and therefore breathe less.

The Respiratory Muscles

Once the message to breathe is sent, it must be carried out. The work of breathing is done by the **respiratory** (or **ventilatory**) **muscles**. The most important ventilatory muscle is the **diaphragm**, which separates the inside of the chest from the abdomen. Since the chest wall (ribs, chest muscles, skin, etc.) is relatively firm, when the diaphragm contracts and moves downward, it leaves more space inside the chest for the lungs to expand. This action causes a vacuum to be formed inside the chest, and air rushes into the trachea and bronchi (through the nose and/or mouth) and fills that extra space. When it is time to breathe out, most of the force comes as the lungs and chest wall just naturally spring back into their usual resting size. With hard breathing, exhalation gets a boost from the expiratory muscles, which include the abdominal muscles, the muscles between the ribs, and some muscles in the neck. During very hard breathing, inhalation gets extra help, too (even the tiny muscles that widen the nostrils contribute to inhalation). All of these muscles are called the **accessory muscles** of respiration, since they are helpful, but are not absolutely necessary for normal quiet breathing. It is possible to see these muscles at work during hard breathing: when the muscles between the ribs (the **intercostal muscles**) are used, the skin seems to sink in between the ribs (this is called *retracting*), and when the neck or abdominal muscles are used, they stick out prominently. If the nose muscles are pitching in, you can see the nostrils widening, a sign called "nasal flaring," or simply "flaring."

Lung Defenses

The air we breathe has an abundance of potentially harmful elements in it (in addition to the good), such as cigarette smoke, pollution, dust, and bacteria and viruses and other germs. And yet, in most people, the lungs stay fairly clean, remaining unclogged by these substances and free from infection. This is the result of a very efficient lung protection system at work.

The Nose and Mouth

The defense of the lungs begins in the nose and mouth. Many of the largest particles breathed in get trapped here, especially in the hairs of the nose.

However, some of the smaller particles do make it past the air conditioning and filtering system of the nose and mouth, and reach the trachea or bronchi. When they reach the bronchi, they get stuck in the mucus that lines the airways. Fortunately, the lung defenses are very active in these lower airways, and can remove small particles through coughing, and the action of the **mucociliary escalator**.

Cough

A cough is an explosive release of air from the lungs. It is something we can do voluntarily, but it can also happen without our conscious control. The steps to producing a cough begin with the stimulation of nerves in the nose, throat, trachea, bronchi, or diaphragm. Some of these nerves can be triggered by pressure, others by noxious chemicals, and others by being touched by inhaled particles. Once the cough signal is sent out, there is a deep breath in, followed by a sudden forcible attempt to breathe out at a time when the upper portion of the airway (around the vocal cords) is tightly shut. Since air cannot get out through this closed door, pressure builds up within the lung. Then, after about one-fifth second, the upper airway suddenly opens and the air bursts out, at a speed reaching 600 miles per hour! This burst of air is very effective in carrying mucus (with its trapped particles of dirt or bacteria) to at least as far as the back of the throat, where it can be spit out or swallowed into the stomach. This tremendous air force is only effective in the largest bronchi and trachea, for the air moves much more slowly in the smaller bronchi farther out in the lungs. Coughing is therefore not an effective method for mucus clearance in the smaller bronchi, and another action is used, which involves the mucociliary escalator.

The Mucociliary Escalator

The trachea and bronchi are lined with little hairs, called **cilia**. Resting atop the cilia is a blanket of mucus, which has been produced by special glands within the bronchi and bronchioles. This layer of mucus protects the airways by trapping substances that might be harmful to the lungs, and removing them through the action of the cilia. The cilia beat approximately 1200 times per minute in a coordinated action that sweeps the mucus (and everything trapped in the mucus) toward the largest bronchi. When the mucus reaches the large central bronchi, it is carried up the trachea in a movement that is similar to that of an escalator. Hence, this system is sometimes referred to as the mucociliary escalator. When the mucus reaches the top of the trachea (the back of the throat) it is swallowed, usually without our being aware of it. This amazing escalator clears about 2 teaspoons of mucus each day. Cigarette smokers and others with extra mucus are often aware of the mucus that has been carried to the back of the throat. If there is an especially large amount, or if it is particularly thick, it may be coughed up once it gets to the large central bronchi. Once it is coughed up, it can be spit out, or it can be swallowed down into the stomach, sending it on its way through the digestive tract, where it will do no harm.

Other Protection Against Lung Infection

Often, bacteria may not be removed immediately, or not completely, by cough or by the mucociliary route. When this happens, further steps are taken to protect the lungs. One such step is the delivery of **white blood cells** to the area where there are foreign substances and bacteria. These blood cells work in two ways: they can release chemicals that attack and destroy the bacteria, and they can also completely surround the bacteria and other particles capturing them within the blood cells. In the latter case, when the blood cell is removed from the lung, the bacteria or other particles are removed also.

There are certain proteins in the blood that also protect the lungs against infection. These are the **immunoglobulins** (gammaglobulin is one such protein). Immunoglobulins are part of a system that recognizes materials that are foreign invaders in all parts of the body, and produces antibodies that attack the foreign substances.

THE RESPIRATORY TRACT IN CYSTIC FIBROSIS

The Upper Respiratory Tract

There are two major differences between the normal upper respiratory tract and that in people with CF. The first difference is in the condition of the **sinuses**, and has very little to do with the person's health or day-to-day comfort. The second difference is the presence of **nasal polyps**, which affects only about 20 percent of people with CF.

The Sinuses

The sinuses of people with CF almost always look abnormal on X-rays. In the X-rays, the sinuses appear as though they are badly diseased, indicating a condition called **pansinusitis** (*-itis* meaning "inflamed," *pan-* meaning "all"; thus, "all the sinuses are inflamed"). It is important to understand the meaning of the appearance of pansinusitis on sinus X-rays for several reasons. First, because it is very unusual to find in children, except in children with CF, the appearance of pansinusitis on the sinus X-rays may help make the diagnosis of CF. Secondly, the appearance of the X-ray will suggest that problems exist such as sinus headaches. However, this is rarely the case. There may be some sinus infection, but this, too, is uncommon. (Sinus infections are discussed in more detail below: *Infections of the Upper Respiratory Tract*.)

At some point a child may have skull X-rays taken, and if the child has CF, the X-rays will most likely show abnormal sinuses. It is important for parents to know that the appearance of sinus abnormality is primarily a problem with the X-ray, that it is not something which bothers the child, and that nothing needs to be done about it.

Typically, treatment is not needed for the sinuses in people with CF. In fact, there is little evidence that sinus surgery is of any use to patients with CF. If a specialist who is not very experienced with CF suggests surgery for the sinuses, a second opinion should be sought. Occasionally, someone with CF may have a sinus infection which actually causes a problem, and antibiotics might then be helpful for the sinuses, but this is relatively uncommon.

The Nose

About 20 percent of CF patients at one time or another will have **nasal polyps**. Polyps are growths of extra tissue that form in various parts of the body. The formation of polyps in the nose occurs much more commonly in CF patients than in people who don't have CF. In fact, this can be another diagnostic clue: if a child has a nasal polyp, this is a strong indication that she or he has CF. Nasal polyps are also found in people who don't have CF, especially in those who have many allergies. In children, however, it is very uncommon to find nasal polyps, except in those with CF.

Generally, having a nasal polyp is not a major problem. It is *never* life-threatening, and it *never* becomes cancerous the way other polyps can in people without CF. What it may do is block up one side of the nose. When there is one polyp, there are often others, and both sides of the nose may become blocked. Rarely, they can become so large that they can protrude from the nostril. In either of these cases (when the polyp blocks the nose or sticks out of the nostril), it is a nuisance but not a threat to the person's health. Since it is usually a significant nuisance at this point, it is advisable to have the polyps removed. One other instance in which it is wise to remove polyps is when, after a period of time, the bridge of the nose grows wider in response to the increasing size of the polyps inside the nose.

It is not yet known why only 20 percent of CF patients get polyps, why most people without CF don't get polyps, or why some CF patients get a polyp once whereas others get them often.

Treatment of nasal polyps

Polyps are strange growths that have a mysterious course of development. They frequently get larger or smaller without treatment, making it difficult to tell if medications are effective. If a polyp gets smaller after medication, one can't be sure that it wouldn't have gotten smaller on its own. Nonetheless, some medications *may* help shrink polyps. These medications are steroid sprays, such as beclomethasone (see *Appendix B: Medications*).

If the medicines don't work, and if the polyp is completely blocking one or both nostrils, or protruding from the nostril, or is widening the outside of the nasal bridge, then surgery to remove the polyp or polyps (*polypectomy*) is advisable. This surgery is best done by an ear, nose, and throat surgeon, in the hospital, and under general anesthesia. In most cases, a very short (overnight) hospital stay is all that is needed. After the surgery, the nose is packed with gauze for several hours to make sure the bleeding has stopped, and once the gauze is removed, the patient can go home. In older patients, the procedure may even be done in the surgeon's office, with local anesthetic. Most often, CF physicians, surgeons, patients, and families feel more comfortable if the surgery is done in the hospital, while the patient is asleep under a general anesthetic.

Surgery is very effective in removing the polyps, and once they are gone, they may never reappear. In some people, though, they may come back, once, twice, or many times.

The Lower Respiratory Tract (the Lungs)

More than any other factor, the lungs determine the health and lifespan of the large majority of patients with CF. In one generation, the greatly improved treatment of the lungs has transformed the outlook for CF infants from one consisting of a few difficult months to one entailing many bright years. Infants with CF are born with lungs that appear normal, but, at varying times after birth, they begin to develop problems. In some, these problems may become noticeable within the first weeks, whereas in others, it may take years or even decades before any problems become apparent. Without treatment, lung problems will eventually appear in anyone with CF and the problems will progress. With treatment, this progression can be slowed, in some, almost to a halt.

The problems start with mucus clogging the smallest airways (the bronchioles), and with subsequent infection and inflammation of those bronchioles (*bronchiolitis*). The inflammation then readily spreads to the larger airways, the bronchi (*bronchitis*). If the mucus is too thick to be cleared by the normal mechanisms, such as the mucociliary escalator, it is very easy for germs (viruses and bacteria) to take hold, which the lungs and body defenses have a difficult time combating.

The more inflammation there is within the bronchi and bronchioles, the more swelling there is (Fig. 1.2), and the narrower the opening becomes to these airways; or, said another way, the greater the bronchial (and bronchiolar) obstruction. With increasing obstruction it becomes more difficult for air to move in and out, which forces the respiratory muscles to work harder. Also, when the airways become obstructed, it is difficult to clear them of mucus. Other mucus-clearing mechanisms, especially cough, are then used

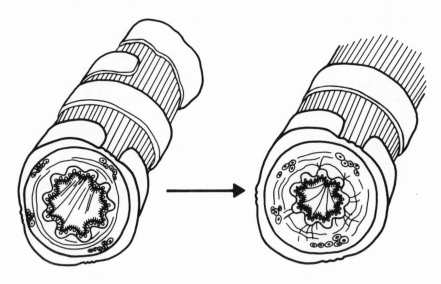

INFLAMMATION MAKES
OPENING NARROW

FIG. 1.2. Inflammation within the bronchi makes the bronchial opening smaller.

more frequently to force the mucus up and out of the bronchioles and bronchi. Increased cough is often the first sign that the bronchial infection and inflammation are getting out of control.

If the bronchial and bronchiolar infection and inflammation remain out of control for too long, they can damage the bronchioles and bronchi, making them enlarged (**dilated**), and weakening their walls so that they become somewhat floppy. The word for abnormal dilatation or distention is *ectasis,* and these changes in the airways are referred to as *bronchiolectasis* and *bronchiectasis.* If the lung damage progresses, it can lead to permanent changes such as infected cysts and scar tissue (*fibrosis*), which are indicated by the name of this disease.

The progression of lung damage is most often very slow and subtle, but it can be relentless. If this progression of infection, inflammation, and lung destruction continues uninterrupted for too long, it will eventually reach a point where there is no longer enough healthy lung to bring oxygen into the body or to eliminate carbon dioxide.

As a particular episode of increased infection and inflammation develops, or as the lung disease increases over the years, the following progression occurs: first, there is more cough. Someone who usually doesn't cough at all may develop a mild cough for a few minutes in the morning, or someone who coughed only in the morning may now cough during the day or through the night. Morning is a common time for people with CF to cough, since they have been in one position for many hours, making it easier for the lung mucus to stay down in the lungs. During the day, when people are active and breathing harder, mucus is more easily shaken loose and sent on its way out of the lungs.

Along with increased cough, there is often a decrease in the ability to exercise, with quicker tiring and even some shortness of breath (difficulty breathing).

As the particular episode of infection and inflammation subsides—on its own or with treatment—the symptoms also subside, either fully or partly, depending on whether any new lung damage has been caused. The goal of treatment is to get back to the baseline (the condition prior to the onset of the problem) after each episode of worsening (*exacerbation*) of lung infection. This is often, but not always, possible.

Asthma

Asthma affects people with or without CF, and is a condition in which the muscles that surround the bronchi squeeze down readily. This ability of the muscles to tighten and make the opening of the bronchi smaller is basically a protective mechanism (see above, *The Airways*), since it can prevent dangerous substances that have been breathed in (*aspirated*) from getting deep into the lungs. But if bronchial wall muscles go into spasm (*bronchospasm*) when there isn't a real threat to the lungs, the end result is that this "protective" mechanism does more harm than good. The bronchi become partly squeezed shut, making it difficult to move mucus out and to breathe air in and out. When the bronchi are narrowed from bronchospasm, there is often a characteristic whistling sound to the breathing. This sound is called *wheezing,* and is heard especially when someone breathes out.

Asthma episodes can be related to allergies, infections, exercise, cold air or to breathing irritating substances such as cigarette smoke or air pollution. In some babies, a condition known as *gastroesophageal reflux* (GE reflux or GER) can also cause bronchospasm (see Chapter 2). Between 10 and 40% of patients with CF also have asthma.

Infections of the Respiratory Tract

This subject can be confusing since there are many different kinds of respiratory infections (which may or may not present serious problems for people with CF), and it is not always clear which are the potentially dangerous ones and which are merely a nuisance.

Infections of the Upper Respiratory Tract

Sinusitis

Sinusitis is an inflammation of the sinuses, usually caused by infection. This is not often a problem for people with CF, even though sinus X-rays always look as though there is an active sinus infection. Many people attribute their cough (or their child's cough) to sinus problems ("mucus drips down my throat and makes me cough"), but this is seldom the case.

Colds

Colds are often referred to as "URI's," for *upper respiratory infections.* Everyone gets colds and has experienced first hand what they are: They are infections of the nose and throat that may involve mucus in the nose, sneezing, and a sore throat. The person with a cold feels generally bad. There may or may not be a fever. Fairly often there is some cough, and scientists don't agree about the cause for the cough. Some say the cough means that there is inflammation in the trachea and bronchi, as well as in the nose and throat, while others say that it results from nose (or sinus) mucus dripping down the back of the throat and tickling the nerves that activate the cough.

Colds are caused by viruses. The main source of cold viruses is other people. People catch colds from other people, who have the cold viruses in their noses and throats. The closer the contact with the infected secretions, the easier it is to catch cold. Sneezing on someone is probably one way to give that person your cold, but the most common way the cold virus is passed around is from one person's respiratory secretions to his or her hand, to the next person's hand, and to that person's mucous membranes in the nose or eyes. Despite what everyone's grandmother has said, *you do not get colds from going out without your galoshes* (or from playing in the snow, or from being outside in cold weather)! In fact, it's probably safer to be outside during cold weather than inside, where there is less ventilation and closer contact with people who might have cold viruses in their noses and on their hands. During the fall and winter seasons, children in day care or school are almost constantly in contact with cold viruses, and are likely to carry those viruses home with them to share with the whole family.

Avoiding colds. Unfortunately, there is little that can be done to avoid catching colds. It is possible to try to avoid colds by staying away from all public places, such as shopping malls, church or temple, and school. However, even this will not be effective in avoiding all contact with the cold viruses. While it is probably sensible to avoid snuggling with someone who has a terrible cold, this also won't do the trick completely since people can have the cold viruses—and pass them on—*before* they feel sick with a cold themselves.

Most colds for people with CF are no worse than colds for other people: You feel miserable, but they do not damage the lungs and they have no long-lasting consequences. Some colds definitely can lead to bronchial infection and can be serious, especially in infants, whose bronchi are tiny and therefore harder to clear of infection. Bronchial infections can be more serious than an infection that stays in the nose and throat, but most often bronchial infections can be successfully treated. In some cases, it may actually be helpful to get a cold. When we are exposed to viruses, our body's immune system produces antibodies that will prevent infections with these same viruses when we are exposed to them at another time. Many infections are more severe later in life, so it's good to get them early and get them over with (mumps and chicken pox are viral infections that are more severe in adults than in children). This doesn't mean that people with CF should try to get as many colds as possible. It just means that it's not worth losing sleep worrying about colds, and no one should disrupt the patient's or family's life in attempting to avoid all colds.

Infections of the Lower Respiratory Tract

Colonization and infection

Most patients with CF have some bacteria in their lungs most of the time (people without CF do not). Whether the bacteria are merely colonizing the lungs (that is, the bacteria are there and have set up colonies, but aren't causing any inflammation or destruction) or whether there is actual infection (that is, bacteria are present and the body has set up an inflammatory reaction to those bacteria, possibly with tissue damage), may be hard to say at any one time.

Bronchiolitis

Bronchiolitis (infection and inflammation of the bronchioles) is most commonly seen during the winter months in babies, with or without CF, and is most often caused by viruses. As many as four babies in 100 without CF will get bronchiolitis in the first 2 years of life. Babies with bronchiolitis may cough and wheeze, become very sick, and need extra oxygen. They may tire to the point of being unable to breathe independently, and require *assisted ventilation,* or *mechanical ventilation.* Both of these terms mean that a machine is used to blow air and oxygen into the baby's lungs. Of course, like any other infection, bronchiolitis can also be a mild disease, with just a little cough and wheezing. Many infants with CF have bronchiolitis as the first sign of a lung problem.

Bronchitis

Bronchitis (infection and inflammation of the bronchi) is a term that is often used incorrectly, referring to a cough that has no obvious cause. Many children and adults with CF have true bronchitis which is caused by bacteria. As was mentioned above, bronchiolitis and bronchitis are the main types of infection that affect the lungs of people with CF. It is these infections that, if not controlled, can lead to lung damage and scarring (fibrosis). Therefore, controlling the episodes of increased infection in the bronchi is the most important part of the treatment of someone with CF. The more lung damage can be prevented or delayed in someone with CF, the better and longer that person's life is likely to be.

Pneumonia

Pneumonia occurs when bacteria, or the blood cells sent to fight bacteria, get into the air sacs (alveoli) or in the lung tissue between the sets of airways. Bacteria and white blood cells are frequently found in these areas in people with CF, but since the infection starts and is mostly confined to the airways, CF lung infections are most accurately thought of as bronchiolitis and bronchitis, and not as pneumonia.

Causes of lung infection in cystic fibrosis

Often it is not clear why a particular lung infection occurs, or why it gets out of control when it does. In some instances it is clear, as, for example, when someone has a cold, and a slight cough that develops into a worse cough remains long after the runny nose has disappeared. In a case such as this, the virus infection that caused this cold has thrown off the balance of the lung defenses enough for some of the hardier bacteria in the lung to multiply and cause problems. In someone who has asthma, the asthma may become worse because of pollution, allergies, cigarette smoke, etc., and lead to a serious infection (it may be difficult in this case to tell how much of the problem is asthma and how much is infection, and which came first). In some cases, there is no explanation of why a lung infection has gotten worse.

Bacteria, viruses, and fungi

Bacteria and viruses are the most important types of germs that cause infection in people with CF; fungi can occasionally cause problems as well.

Bacteria. Bacteria are probably the major cause of bronchial infection (and lung damage) in people with CF. Bacteria are larger than viruses, and can usually be killed by antibiotics. Normally, the number of bacteria in the lungs of someone with CF is relatively small, and the body's defenses (immune system) are able to keep these bacteria under control. But when something happens to offset this balance, the bacteria can multiply and cause inflammation. In this situation, there is bronchial infection and not just colonization.

The bacteria that most often colonize and infect the lungs of people with CF are *Haemophilus influenzae,* sometimes called H. flu (not to be confused with the influenza virus); *Staphylococcus,* or "staph"; and *Pseudomonas aeruginosa.* Other bacteria that can be found include *Klebsiella, E. coli, Serratia, Pseudomonas maltophilia,* and *Pseudomonas cepacia. Streptococcus,* which causes strep throat, and *Pneumococcus,* sometimes called the "pneumonia germ" because it is the most common cause of pneumonia in people with normal lungs, are not especially common in people with CF.

The most prevalent bacteria affecting people are probably staph and the various types of *Pseudomonas.* The *Pseudomonas* family has a reputation, which is only partially deserved, of being particularly dangerous bacteria. Though it is harder to kill than other bacteria—especially with antibiotics that are taken by mouth—it is *not* true that *Pseudomonas* (or any other particular bacteria) is the kiss of death. The important factor is not *what bacteria* are in the lung, but rather *what harm* they are causing. Many people with CF have *Pseudomonas* colonization of the bronchi for many years and experience little or no trouble. If someone has no cough, no problems exercising, and no trouble breathing, it doesn't much matter if a throat or mucus culture has shown *Pseudomonas.* On the other hand, if someone does have all those problems, and the culture grows only staph, the person is still sick.

Recently, it appeared that *Pseudomonas cepacia* was an especially dangerous form of *Pseudomonas,* causing death shortly after colonization. It now seems that this is not always the case, and that some types of *Pseudo-monas cepacia* are no worse than other *Pseudomonas*. The major issue is how much damage they cause, and how readily they are killed by antibiotics.

Viruses. Viruses are smaller than bacteria, and generally cannot be killed by medicines. Antibiotics have no effect on viruses. Viruses are the most common cause of upper respiratory infections (colds), and may affect the bronchi as well. Some of the common respiratory viruses are respiratory syncytial virus (RSV), parainfluenza virus, rhinovirus, and influenza virus. This last virus, influenza ("flu"), causes epidemics in the winter, afflicting many people with miserable cold-like symptoms. Influenza can cause a very serious pneumonia which can even be fatal.

Some of the common childhood illnesses, such as chicken pox, measles, mumps, and rubella (German measles), are caused by viruses. On rare occasions, measles can cause a very serious pneumonia. This is true of chicken pox (varicella) as well, although most CF experts feel that this is unlikely in someone with CF.

Fungi. Fungi, especially the fungus *Aspergillus fumigatus,* are sometimes found in the bronchi of CF patients. They can cause trouble, but not usually in the same way as viruses or bacteria. The problem with *Aspergillus* is not infection with tissue damage, but rather an allergic reaction (*allergic bron-chopulmonary aspergillosis,* or ABPA), which induces swelling within the bronchi.

Treatment of the Lungs in Cystic Fibrosis

Since the main problems in the lungs are obstruction of bronchioles and bronchi and the resulting infection, treatment is aimed at both relieving bron-chial blockage and fighting infection.

Relieving and Preventing Obstruction

Chest physical therapy

A major portion of most treatment programs is aimed at keeping the air-ways as free of mucus as possible. The methods seem crude, but are quite effective and are based on a principle taken from everyday life, namely, the "Ketchup Bottle Principle": If you want to get a thick substance out of a container with a narrow opening, you turn the container upside down so that its opening is pointing downward, and then you clap it, shake it, and vibrate it. If the thick substance is mucus, and the container is the various segments of the lungs, the procedure is the same, and may be equally effective: you turn the child (or yourself) in various positions, with each position allowing one of the major portions of the lungs to have its opening pointing downward, and then you clap firmly on the back or chest over that part of the lung, and actually shake the mucus loose. Once it's shaken loose, the mucus can fall into the large central airways, and then be coughed out. This form of treatment goes by many different names, a few of which are postural drainage (PD's), chest physical therapy (chest PT, or just CPT), and percussion and drainage. Often, children and families invent their own pet names: "exercises," "clapping," "boom-booms."

PD treatments are not painful; in fact, they can be very soothing and relaxing in the way that a massage is. Babies who may be crying at the beginning of their PD's are often asleep halfway through the procedure. The treatment can be time-consuming, however (from 1 to 2 minutes for each of 10 or 12 positions), and can be a bother to children, adolescents, and adults alike since it interferes with the day's agenda. It may also keep an older child or adult tied to home, since it is awkward to perform on oneself and may require accommodating to someone else's (usually a parent's) schedule.

There are several pieces of equipment that make these treatments easier to perform at home. The first is the mechanical percussor/vibrator. This tool comes in a variety of models, the simplest of which is like an electric jigsaw that has a rod with a firm cushion on it. The cushion is held on the chest and bounces firmly and repeatedly where it is aimed. Most models have variable force and speed; some models are driven by electricity and others by compressed air. The action of some models is a pounding motion whereas others vibrate; some models can do both, depending on the setting selected. Treatments with the good mechanical percussors are probably just as effective as those done by hand, if conscientiously performed. Some children (and adults, too) have a strong preference for the hand, whereas others prefer the machines. Clearly, a treatment by either method is considerably more effective than no treatment at all.

The mechanical devices have two advantages over the manual method. Most of the mechanical percussors or vibrators come with extension handles or straps, which enable teenagers or adults to reach areas of the back that they could not reach by hand. This makes it possible for them to give themselves a full treatment independently. Another advantage of the mechanical percussors is that they are gentler on the elbow and shoulder joints of the person who performs the treatments—a great advantage for a parent who has more than one child requiring treatment each day.

Another device that simplifies treatment is a PD table. Treatments for infants and small children are done most comfortably with the child on a parent's lap, but when the patient is an adolescent or an adult the table becomes very useful. The person receiving the treatment can sit or lie on the table, which can be set at different angles, thereby making proper positioning easier to achieve. Tables and percussors can be bought from commercial suppliers, but since many centers have tables available for no charge (supplied by charitable organizations), it is worth checking with your CF center before you purchase one.

Exercise

Many people believe that vigorous exercise may be helpful to loosen mucus and to keep bronchi clear. Certainly, hard exercise, or laughing or crying, often result in a coughing spell that brings up mucus, even in people who do not raise mucus during the traditional PD treatments. Since there is not yet any scientific evidence that exercise can successfully replace the time-honored PD treatments, it is best to encourage patients to be very active *and* to do their treatments.

One point to keep in mind is that a method may be helpful even if it does not result in the immediate expectoration of large amounts of mucus. Mucus might be shaken loose from the smallest bronchioles and started on its way to the central bronchi, but it will not cause a cough until it actually reaches the large, central bronchi. There is good evidence that regular PD's are helpful, even though a single treatment makes little or no apparent difference. In one study, a number of children stopped their PD's for 3 weeks, and had a significant deterioration in their lung function (even though they didn't *feel* any different); when they resumed their treatments after the 3-week experimental period, their lung function returned to its previous level.

Other methods of clearing mucus

A number of other procedures that rely upon forcible exhalation ("huff") have been employed to increase mucus clearance. Breathing out hard through a tube or face mask with a narrow opening is one such method. While these methods are relatively new, they may prove to be helpful.

Breaking up mucus

Can adding water to the mucus in airways make the mucus more watery and easier to cough out? This idea seems to make sense, but there is no evidence that inhaling water can make the mucus thinner. One medication, acetylcysteine (Mucomyst), is inhaled as an aerosol by many people with CF to break up mucus. When Mucomyst is mixed with CF mucus in a test tube, it does make the mucus thinner and easier to move. However, human bronchi and tracheas are different from glass test tubes, and may react with inflammation when Mucomyst is inhaled. Some people have developed increasing bronchial obstruction because of inflammation, or even bronchospasm, after inhaling Mucomyst. While some people do improve with this treatment, most are neither helped nor hurt by it.

Treating asthma

When asthma is present in addition to CF, there is increased bronchial obstruction with which to contend. Bronchospasm makes the opening of the bronchi smaller than normal, making it much more difficult to get the mucus out. Several very effective bronchodilator medications, which dilate (open)

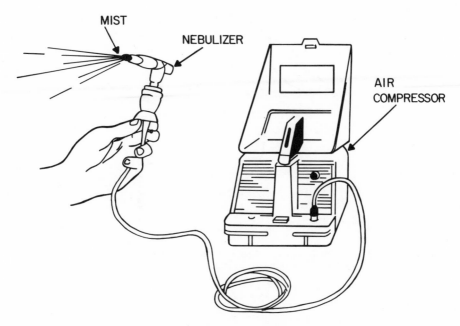

MIST

NEBULIZER

AIR COMPRESSOR

FIG. 1.3. Aerosol machine. The machine blows compressed air through the tubing, creating a mist from the liquid medication. The patient then breathes the medicine.

the bronchi are available. These medications can be inhaled, as an aerosol, or taken by mouth or injection. The aerosols are delivered by an aerosol machine, which is composed of an air compressor, a length of tubing, and a nebulizer (Fig. 1.3). The compressor sends air through the tube to the nebulizer, which holds the liquid medicine. As the air rushes by, it lifts the medicine, breaks it into a mist, and blows it out through the mouthpiece or mask to be inhaled. Some medications are available in hand-held metered-dose inhalers (Fig. 1.4). These devices deliver a measured amount of medicated mist with each puff. Since the puff of medicine is only available for breathing in for a fraction of a second, the timing of the puffing and breathing in is crucial, and may be quite difficult to coordinate, especially for small children. Extension devices are now available which attach to the opening of the inhaler and make the timing less crucial. Some aerosol bronchodilator medications are metaproterenol (Alupent, Metaprel), isoetharine (Bronkosol), and albuterol (Ventolin, Proventil) (see *Appendix B: Medications*).

Oral bronchodilators include some of the same medications that are inhaled. These are all in the family of *beta-adrenergic* drugs (metaproterenol, albuterol). Another family of bronchodilators that can be taken by mouth are the theophyllines. Theophylline is related to caffeine, which is actually a weak bronchodilator. Theophylline comes in the form of a liquid, tablet, or capsule (fast-acting or sustained-release) (see *Appendix B: Medications*).

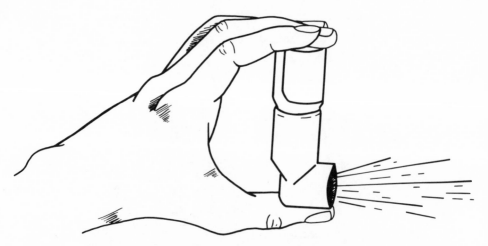

FIG. 1.4. Hand-held nebulizer (also called metered-dose inhaler). Pushing down the top of the inhaler causes a puff of medicated mist to shoot out into the air, for the patient to breathe in.

Reducing airway inflammation

Airway inflammation often accompanies infection and/or asthma (see above, *The Lower Respiratory Tract*), making the airway opening that much smaller. Some medications, most notably a group of drugs called *steroids,* can reduce inflammation wherever it occurs, including in the bronchial tree. Within the past few years, prednisone (one of the steroids) has been used by a limited number of people with CF, and has appeared to be effective in improving their lung function.

The assumption behind the use of prednisone in people with CF is that when their immune system responds to infection in the bronchi, it does so with an excess of inflammation. Although inflammation is a normal part of fighting infection (see above, *Other Protection Against Lung Infection*), if it gets out of control it can do more harm than good. Prednisone inhibits this overactive response, thereby reducing the swelling within the airways and making the patients better.

Prednisone, however, is a very potent drug that has many possible side effects (see *Appendix B: Medications*). One of the most serious of these side effects is *over*suppression of the immune response, which makes the body unable to fight infection. Because of these and other possible side effects, most CF physicians have wanted to see more studies of the benefits and dangers of prednisone before prescribing it on a regular basis for their patients. If the medication is given on alternate days (as was done in one study), the chances of dangerous side effects are much less, but still not entirely absent.

There are other drugs that reduce inflammation without interfering with the body's ability to fight infection. These drugs include aspirin and related drugs, which are used for people with arthritis. While they might be able to provide the benefits of prednisone without the dangers, they have their own problems as well. Studies are currently being conducted that examine the risks and the benefits of these various approaches to inflammation.

Reducing Bronchial Infection

Antibacterial drugs (antibiotics)

These drugs are probably the most important single factor responsible for the tremendous improvement in the outlook for people with CF, both in terms of length of life and quality of life. Antibiotics are very effective in reducing airways infection, and therefore in preserving lung health. (See *Appendix B: Medications* for a more complete discussion of antibiotics.) Most CF physicians agree that antibiotics should be used when there is evidence of increased airways infection (such as increased cough and mucus production and decreased exercise tolerance). There is no agreement, however, on whether it is helpful to give antibiotics on a regular basis to *prevent* infection.

Oral antibiotics are usually taken when the infection is caused by staph or *Hemophilus*. (See Appendix B for a review of these antibiotics.) Oral antibiotics may, on occasion, be helpful for *Pseudomonas* infections, but most often they will not bring these infections under control. If this is the case, someone may need treatment with intravenous antibiotics, which usually requires a hospital stay (see Chapter 5). Some antibiotics can be given by aerosol.

Preventing bacterial infection

There is no very effective method for preventing bronchial infections caused by bacteria. There is, however, a vaccine available that is moderately good at preventing infection with the *Pneumococcus* bacteria. Since this is the most common cause of pneumonia in the general population, the vaccine is often called "the pneumonia vaccine." People who are at risk from pneumonia, such as the elderly and people with sickle cell disease, are encouraged to get this vaccine. Since people with CF are not very likely to get pneumococcal pneumonia, or if they get it they do not usually have trouble getting rid of it, there is no particular need for them to get the "pneumonia vaccine."

Fighting viral infections

There are very few safe drugs that kill viruses, and, therefore, no safe, effective drug treatment for viral bronchiolitis or bronchitis. One exception is ribavirin, which seems to be effective for very sick babies with bronchiolitis caused by the respiratory syncytial virus (RSV). This drug is delivered by an aerosol, and must be breathed in for as long as 12 hours at a time. Ribavirin is not effective for infections caused by most other viruses, and specifically, it provides little benefit to people with colds.

One other exception is amantadine, which appears to be helpful in fighting the influenza virus. It is taken by mouth, and is used primarily by people who become infected with influenza during an epidemic. People who are at risk for influenza infection, such as CF patients who have not had the flu vaccine, may also take the drug as a preventive measure, during a community outbreak of influenza.

Preventing viral infections

The most common type of viral infection, namely, the common cold, cannot be effectively prevented (see above, *Infections of the Upper Respiratory Tract*). There are other viral infections that *can* be prevented, though, including measles and influenza ("flu"). All children should be immunized against measles, and all children with CF (or other abnormal lung conditions) should receive a flu shot each year. These vaccines are effective and are safe except in people with very severe egg allergy.

Zoster immune globulin, or ZIG, is a gammaglobulin-like shot that is given to prevent chicken pox. Most CF physicians feel, however, that this is unnecessary for people with CF, since the chances that someone with CF would have lung complications from chicken pox are very small. In addition, a major drawback to ZIG is that once it is given, it has to be repeated every time there is an exposure to chicken pox. Nonetheless, some CF physicians recommend ZIG for patients who have been exposed to chicken pox. Others recommend "chicken pox parties" for children who have not yet had chicken pox. In this way, they will come in contact with a "poxy" child and contract chicken pox in childhood when it's likely to be mild, instead of in adulthood when it often follows a much more severe course.

Steps to Treating Worsened Lungs

It is the nature of CF for the lungs to get worse from time to time. These periods of worsening, called *pulmonary exacerbations,* are most often caused by increased airways infection, and can usually be brought under control if proper steps are taken.

Recognition

In order for pulmonary exacerbations to be treated, they must first be recognized, which is not always easy. The signs that the lungs are worse may be very subtle, and may at first escape attention. These signs include more cough than usual, more mucus, decreased energy, poor appetite, difficulty exercising, and shortness of breath. In most people, the amount of cough is the single most important clue. Many people will *not* have lessened activity or shortness of breath, nor will they have fever, so the absence of these clues should not be taken as a reassuring sign. It is important to recognize when there are more signs of infection than are usual for *you*, since everyone is different. For example, if your usual pattern is to cough only a little bit in the morning, but you begin to cough after laughing or crying and find that the cough lasts just a bit longer, then you will know that your condition is not quite as good as it usually is. On occasion, someone else, such as your doctor or a relative who doesn't see you every day, may point a difference out to you that you haven't observed. Sometimes, however, it may take an X-ray or pulmonary function test to show that a change has occurred. For this reason, it is quite important to make fairly frequent clinic visits. It's very tempting to say, "I [or my child] am doing so well that there's no need to go for a checkup." There are far too many CF patients (usually teenagers) and parents of patients who have used this reasoning, only to return to regular care after irreversible lung damage has been done. Regular visits, which would include physical examinations, throat or sputum cultures, and periodic chest X-rays and pulmonary function tests, can often spot a problem while it is still reversible. Since the progression of lung disease in CF is usually very gradual and subtle—and is *not* characterized by sudden dramatic deterioration—it is easy for patients and families to miss signs of deterioration. Your physician may be able to recognize these signs, because a change in the weeks or months since your last visit is easier to detect than small day-to-day changes, and because sensitive laboratory tests (pulmonary function tests and X-rays) help clarify your condition.

Once you have recognized that there is a problem, it is important not to wait until you're terribly ill to do something about it. That wait can give the infection and inflammation an opportunity to destroy a small portion of lung, leaving a little scar tissue behind. Scar tissue can never become normal lung tissue, so it's important to prevent its formation.

Oral and aerosol antibiotics

During a period of worsening, your physician will probably prescribe an oral antibiotic, or change the antibiotic if you are already taking one. The choice of antibiotics is based on several factors, including how the individual patient has responded in the past, how sick the person is at the time, and what recent throat or sputum cultures have shown (what bacteria are there and which antibiotics kill those bacteria in the lab). The physician may also increase the number of PD treatments you're doing, in order to clear out the extra mucus that builds up with infections.

If an infection does not improve quickly, and certainly if it becomes worse, it is advisable to take the next step of changing antibiotics. This change will

be to a more powerful antibiotic, or to one that is better at killing the particular bacteria a culture has shown to be in your system. If a more powerful
or appropriate oral antibiotic is not available, or if the physician feels that
an oral antibiotic would work too slowly, then he or she may recommend an
aerosol antibiotic.

Intravenous antibiotics

If these steps do not work, or do not work fast enough, it may be time for
intravenous (IV) antibiotics. In almost every case, putting antibiotics into a
vein is the most effective way of treating infection, especially if the infection
is caused by *Pseudomonas*. Typically, the administration of IV antibiotics
requires a hospital stay. In some cases, it is possible to get IV's at home.
(For more information about IV's and hospitalization, see Chapter 5.)

The length of time to give IV antibiotics should be determined by how the
patient is responding to treatment. Patients seldom improve (and may perhaps even worsen) in the first 4 or 5 days on IV's. Thereafter, most people
improve for several weeks, then return to their usual condition or even to an
improved condition. On occasion, someone may stop improving without
having returned to his or her previous baseline. Studies have shown that the
level of lung function achieved after in-hospital IV treatment of a pulmonary

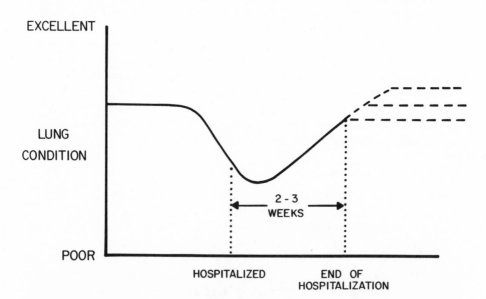

FIG. 1.5. Timing of hospitalization. When it is recognized that the patient is not doing well
out of the hospital, he or she is admitted to the hospital for treatment. Improvement begins
within several days. Hospital treatment then continues until the patient has gotten back to
his or her usual state of health.

exacerbation can be maintained for at least several weeks, but will not continue to improve after discharge from the hospital. Therefore, it makes sense to get the most mileage possible from the IV and hospital treatment, and not to stop after a predetermined number of days have gone by. Some people will have gotten the maximum benefit from the intensive treatment in as short a time as 10 days, but most people take about 2 weeks, and quite a few people take even longer. Keep in mind that this investment of time can pay off in the long run if it keeps even a small portion of lung from becoming scarred. Figure 1.5 shows a time curve for when someone should enter the hospital, and when he or she should leave.

Other treatments

In some cases, other treatments may be used with IV antibiotics or tried before them. One example is trying medications to decrease bronchial inflammation, like prednisone. Another example is altering antiasthma medications by increasing their dosage, or by adding different ones. The best steps to take will differ under different conditions.

Complications

There are several problems that can be an indirect result of CF. These problems are often referred to as *complications* of CF. The most important complications related to the lung disease of CF are hemoptysis, atelectasis, pneumothorax, respiratory failure, heart failure, and chest pain. Other complications which relate to the lung disease of CF affect the bones and/or the joints.

Hemoptysis

The literal translation of this term is to "cough up blood" (*heme* is the Greek word for "blood," and *ptyein* translates as "to spit"). Hemoptysis is very uncommon in young children with CF, but as many as 50 percent of adults with CF will on occasion have some streaks of blood in the mucus they cough up and spit out. A relatively small proportion of patients (about 3–5 percent of those older than 15 years) will cough out large (more than 10 ounces) amounts of blood at a time. This problem, called *massive hemoptysis,* can be fatal, although it rarely is, even in people who bring up very large amounts of blood. In most cases, the significance of hemoptysis is the same as that of an increased cough, namely, both are signs of increased infection. A major difference, however, between having a bit more cough than usual and bringing up bright red blood is that it is very frightening to see the blood, especially the first time it happens. One's first reaction is to panic and to assume that all of one's lungs must be bleeding. This is not the case:

It's extremely important to know that *hemoptysis is a fairly common problem that is almost always simple to treat.*

What is happening is that the increased infection in one small area has irritated a capillary or small artery and made a small hole in its wall, causing blood to leak out into the airway. Remember that the size of the working surface of the lungs is about the same as a tennis court; the problem area in someone with hemoptysis is about the size of a little pebble on that tennis court. It helps to keep this in mind if you should see some blood mixed in with mucus sometime. If you see *pure* blood, you should notify your doctor, because you do need treatment, but there's no need to panic.

In unusual cases, hemoptysis can mean something other than just increased infection. It can indicate a more general bleeding problem. Bleeding problems can be caused by inadequate vitamin K (this would be uncommon in someone with CF who is getting a good diet and taking the prescribed enzymes), by advanced liver disease, or rarely by a drug side effect. In some unusual situations it may be difficult to tell where spit-up blood has come from. Bleeding in the stomach or esophagus can be confused with bleeding in the lungs. Fortunately, bleeding in the stomach or esophagus is not common in people with CF.

Treating hemoptysis

The treatment required for someone who coughs up bloody mucus, or pure blood, depends on the cause of the bleeding. In most cases, the cause is an increase in bronchial infection which has irritated a blood vessel, and the treatment therefore is the same as the treatment for any increased infection, namely, antibiotics and PD treatments. There is little or no controversy about the need for antibiotics (or for stronger antibiotics in someone who is already taking antibiotics). Not all CF specialists agree on the usefulness of PD, and, in fact, some experts recommend stopping PD treatments in someone who has brought up a large amount of blood. However, in most cases, the clapping and vibrating are very unlikely to cause any bleeding and should be continued.

In some people who bring up blood, a gurgling sensation is felt in the chest (they can sometimes even tell which part of the lung it's coming from) just before the blood comes up. If someone feels a gurgling every time he or she goes into a particular position, the head-down position, for example, then that position should be avoided. In general, though, the treatments should be continued as much as possible, for three reasons: (1) the blood is not good for cilia and should therefore be removed; (2) the blood can make an infection worse by providing a hospitable environment for bacteria; and (3) even if the blood itself is not a problem, one of the underlying principles of treating bronchial infection in someone with CF is to lessen bronchial mucous obstruction as much as possible.

In most cases where a person has brought up a large amount (more than a cup) of pure blood, hospitalization is recommended. In the hospital, IV antibiotics can be given easily, and patients can be watched carefully to make sure the bleeding is under control. If the bleeding is very severe and much blood has been lost, blood transfusions may be necessary, just as they would be if the bleeding were caused by a car accident, for example. It is quite uncommon, however, for a transfusion to be required.

Extra vitamin K is usually given to someone with CF who has hemoptysis, since a lack of that vitamin can cause bleeding problems. If the bleeding is not controlled fairly quickly it may be necessary to do various tests. These tests would check for a generalized bleeding problem (as might occur in someone with severe liver disease) or examine the possibility that the bleeding is a side effect of a drug or drug combination.

In a few cases of massive hemoptysis that can't be controlled by the above means, more difficult methods may be needed. One such method is *bronchoscopy,* which allows the physician to look into the lungs with a flexible tube that goes through the nose and down the back of the throat, or with a rigid tube that is passed directly down the throat. Most physicians, however, doubt that bronchoscopy is very helpful, and a relatively new procedure is more likely to be recommended. This procedure is called *bronchial artery embolization,* and has been helpful in people with massive hemoptysis. An *embolus* is a clot or other plug in a blood vessel that blocks the circulation in that vessel (*embolos* is the Greek word for "plug"). Emboli are usually harmful, but they can also be helpful when a bronchial artery is leaking. In this case, a radiologist may be able to thread a catheter (a thin, flexible tube) into the artery and inject a plug (typically made of a synthetic substance called Gelfoam) through the catheter that will then seal the leak and stop the bleeding.

There are several problems that make this procedure less than perfect. The first is that it is not always possible to find the artery that is leaking, even with the sophisticated radiologic technology that is available. The second problem is that, in some people, arteries to the spinal cord may come from the bronchial arteries. If the Gelfoam plug blocks off the blood supply to a portion of the spinal cord, serious problems could result. Fortunately, with modern techniques, the radiologist can nearly always tell beforehand if the patient has such a spinal artery, and can plan the plugging accordingly. Lastly, a fair proportion of people whose bleeding has been stopped with bronchial artery embolization will bleed again from that spot in the future.

In a very few cases—when there is massive bleeding and bronchial artery embolization cannot be performed or is not successful—surgery may be necessary to remove the lobe of the lung that is the source of the bleeding. There are numerous problems with this approach, a major one being that, although the person will obviously not bleed again from the removed lobe, he or she will also not have the use of that lobe for breathing. In addition, general anesthesia and chest surgery carry their own risks, especially in someone with severe lung disease. Finally, even with the chest open, it may not be possible to identify the lobe that is the source of bleeding with absolute certainty. There are too many cases of CF patients who have had a lobe removed in a hospital inexperienced in CF care, only to be transferred to a CF center because the bleeding didn't stop. Nonetheless, there *are* some cases in which surgery is necessary and very successful.

Because of the problems and uncertainties with the invasive means of dealing with hemoptysis, many CF experts prefer to treat patients—even those with massive hemoptysis—as conservatively as possible, with antibiotics, PD, vitamin K, transfusions if necessary, and careful observation.

Pneumothorax

This complication is also called "collapsed lung." The term actually means "air inside the chest," which doesn't sound all that abnormal, since that's where air is supposed to be. But it actually refers to air that's within the chest, but *outside the lung* (Fig. 1.6). That is very abnormal, and can be dangerous, since once air gets outside the lung, it can press in on it and cause it to collapse. If there is enough air under enough pressure or tension, it can even squeeze the blood vessels (venae cavae) that bring the blood back to the heart. This will mean that there won't be enough blood to pump out to the body to keep it functioning normally. This does not usually happen with a pneumothorax in someone with CF. It is unusual for pneumothorax to occur in someone under the age of 10, and after age 10, between 10 and 25 percent of CF patients will develop a pneumothorax. Pneumothorax is much more likely to happen in someone with CF if there is relatively severe lung involvement than if the lungs are in very good shape.

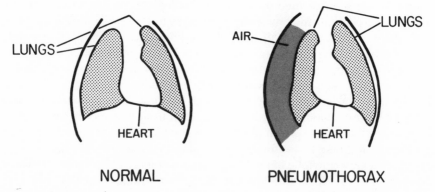

FIG. 1.6. X-ray appearance of pneumothorax. The air outside of the lung appears black, while the lungs are gray.

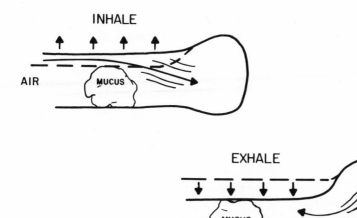

FIG. 1.7. Partial obstruction of bronchi may cause progressive overinflation of a portion of lung, leading to pneumothorax. The bronchi enlarge slightly when one inhales, allowing air to get into the lungs past the mucus. When one exhales, the bronchi get smaller, trapping the air behind the blockage. With each breath, more and more air can become trapped, leading to progressive overinflation, and eventual tearing of the tissue allowing air to escape from the lung.

Pneumothorax develops when mucus partially blocks a bronchus or bronchiole, and functions as a one-way valve or "ball-valve" (Fig. 1.7). This kind of blockage allows air to go in only one direction past the blockage. Bronchi enlarge with inhaling, and get smaller with exhaling (see *The Airways*). When mucus fills up a portion of a bronchiole, the bronchiole will enlarge enough with each breath that some air can get beyond the mucous plug. But during exhaling, the bronchus may collapse to the same size as the plug, so no air will escape. When this happens, the alveoli beyond the blockage will get bigger with each breath in, until, like an overfilled balloon, they finally burst. If these overfilled alveoli are at the edge of the lung (especially at the apex, or top, of the lung), when they burst, the air leaks out of the lung.

A pneumothorax almost always causes sudden sharp pain in the chest, side, or back, and difficulty breathing (shortness of breath). The only way to tell for certain if someone has a pneumothorax is with a chest X-ray. The X-ray will show an area inside the chest that is completely black, rather than the usual combination of white and gray; there will also be a clear outline to the edge of the collapsed lung. Some people "score" pneumothoraces on the basis of how much of the lung is collapsed on the X-ray. A "25 percent pneumothorax" means that air outside the lung takes up 25 percent of the space that the lung normally occupies, and that the lung itself has collapsed to 75 percent of its normal size. If someone with relatively healthy lungs develops a pneumothorax, this can be a useful description. But when a pneumothorax occurs in someone with CF, it's less helpful, since the lungs tend to be stiff in people with CF, and therefore may not collapse readily, even with quite a bit of air outside, under quite a bit of tension. So, what looks like a small amount of air may actually be a lot.

Since pneumothoraces need to be treated, you should let your doctor know if you ever develop sudden chest pain and shortness of breath.

Treatment of pneumothorax

The treatment for pneumothorax usually requires hospitalization, and is directed toward accomplishing three goals: (1) relieving the pressure on the lung by evacuating the air from around the lung, (2) sealing over the hole through which the air has escaped, and (3) ideally, preventing recurrence. There are rare instances in which there is a tiny pneumothorax—just the smallest bit of air outside the lung, with the leak already sealed off by itself— and no treatment is needed. Much more commonly, if there is a pneumothorax, all three treatment goals should be met.

The pressure is usually relieved by a chest tube. This is a tube that goes through the skin, between the ribs, and into the pleural space, which is the space between the chest wall and the outside of the lung. This is the space where air accumulates if it leaks out of the lung. The tube is hooked up to a vacuum that sucks the air out continuously and allows the lung to expand to its normal size. The system of tubing used to evacuate the air from the pleural space must have a good valving system (most often provided by having the tubes pass through a series of vacuum jars or a water seal) so that air can pass only out of the chest, and not back into it. The physician makes a small skin incision to place the chest tube, then pushes the tube into place and hooks up the vacuum. Placement of the tube can be painful, and having a tube in place is also uncomfortable. If the treatment chosen is only chest tube placement, the treatment is often successful in the short run, but very unsuccessful in the long run. Most air leaks will seal themselves eventually, so a chest tube can evacuate the air, and sooner or later the air will stop accumulating, so the tube can be pulled out. Unfortunately, it may take many days for this self-sealing to occur, and during this time, the painful chest tube will interfere with the deep breathing and coughing needed to keep the lungs clear. Even when the leak does seal itself, between 50 and 100 percent of these pneumothoraces will recur unless further steps are taken to prevent this from happening.

There are two main approaches to sealing the leak and preventing recurrences of pneumothorax. Both approaches purposely cause inflammation of the pleural surface (the covering of the lung), almost like a burn, so that when the irritated surfaces heal, the healing scar tissue will cover over any weak, leaky area. The first approach is called *chemical sclerosing* or *chem-*

ical pleurodesis. For this method, it is necessary to have a chest tube in the pleural space (the space between the lung and the chest wall). An irritating chemical (such as tetracycline, talc, or quinicrine) is sent through the tube once a day for three days in a row. When the chemical is pushed through the tube, the patient rotates through different positions, holding each one for several minutes in order to distribute the chemical to all surfaces of the lungs. The head-down position is particularly important, since the weakest spots are usually at the apex (top) of the lung. If the treatment is successful, it causes intense inflammation, and therefore is often very painful. Pain medication prior to the daily procedure is essential.

Another method of causing inflammation of the surface of the lung is with a surgical operation, during which the patient is asleep under general anesthesia. The surgeon makes an incision between the ribs, spreads the ribs, and examines the lung for weak spots ("blebs"). These areas are then cut out, and the remaining hole is sewn closed. The next step is to strip the pleura off the upper part of the lung, which leaves the lung surface irritated. The side and lower portions of the lung are more difficult to strip of their pleural covering, so the surgeon will take a piece of gauze and rub the surface roughly to set up the same kind of irritation and inflammation. (This whole procedure is referred to as *open thoracotomy, apical pleurectomy, and pleurabrasion,* which means "cutting the chest open, stripping the membrane off the uppermost portion of the lung, and rubbing the rest of the lung surface.")

When the chest is closed, a chest tube must be left in to drain the extra air outside the lung. Usually that tube can come out when the air has been fully evacuated, and when it is clear that the leaks have been sealed. Although this procedure sounds brutal, the patient is asleep and feels no pain. After the surgery, the main discomfort is from the chest tube, which is usually removed within a few days. It is surprising, but true, that most people have less discomfort with the surgical treatment than with the chemical sclerosing. This treatment by an experienced surgeon is nearly 100 percent successful in preventing recurrences of pneumothorax in the involved lung.

Atelectasis

This term is derived from two Greek words (*ateles* + *ektasis*), meaning "incomplete" and "expansion," and refers to different kinds of incomplete expansion of the lung or part of the lung. Atelectasis is also a kind of collapsed lung, but is very different from a pneumothorax. In someone with CF, atelectasis is almost always caused by mucus which completely blocks a bronchus leading to one of the lobes or segments of a lung (much more often in the right lung than the left, and more often in the upper lobe than in other lobes). If the opening to a lobe or segment is blocked, air cannot get into that portion of the lung. Eventually all the air that was in that lobe or

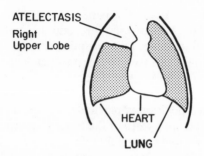

ATELECTASIS
Right
Upper Lobe

HEART

LUNG

FIG. 1.8. X-ray appearance of atelectasis. The portion of the lung that does not contain air (the atelectatic portion) appears white, while the rest of the lung is gray.

segment gets absorbed, leaving the lobe or segment airless. On an X-ray it will appear white (solid) instead of the usual combination of white and gray (Fig. 1.8). About one of every 20 people with CF will develop atelectasis at some point. This problem is more common in infants than older people, probably because their bronchi are smaller and therefore more readily blocked. Usually, atelectasis does not cause any specific signs or symptoms, but is likely to occur during a period of worsened lung infection.

Treating atelectasis

Since atelectasis occurs when mucus totally blocks the opening of the bronchi in a segment or lobe of a lung, the treatment is similar to the maintenance care designed to keep the bronchi clear on a regular basis. The mainstay of the treatment is PD and percussion. Once atelectasis is identified, the physician will recommend increasing the frequency of PD treatments, perhaps to as often as four times a day. Most physicians will also recommend antibiotics, since infection may have caused the bronchial obstruction (by generating more mucus), and may also result from the obstruction. Physicians who don't usually advise their patients to inhale mucus-cutting drugs such as Mucomyst (see *Appendix B: Medications*) may make an exception in treating atelectasis. There is little or no information to support its use, however.

Bronchoscopy (see above, *Hemoptysis*) with *lavage* (washing out mucus from the bronchi) is often employed in treating atelectasis. This is an appealing kind of treatment based on the logic that if mucus is blocking the bronchi, why not just go in and wash it out? Though it is logical, this treatment, unfortunately, is rarely successful.

The most inclusive study to examine the results of treating atelectasis with many different methods has shown that the traditional methods of PD and antibiotics are just as successful as invasive methods such as bronchoscopy. Successful treatment of atelectasis, regardless of the method chosen, may be slow, and it may take weeks or even months before the condition responds to treatment.

Low Oxygen Level

Most people with CF who have any more than the mildest amount of lung disease will have a lower-than-normal blood oxygen level. In most cases, this causes no problems. If someone lives at sea level, extra oxygen is needed only when the lung disease is very severe. At higher altitudes, the air pressure is so low that it's harder to move oxygen from the air in the alveoli into the bloodstream. At the top of Mount Everest, the air pressure is less than half of what it is at sea level; up there, *everyone* needs to breathe extra oxygen. In Denver (and in the passenger cabins of commercial airliners), the pressure is about four-fifths of the sea level pressure. For people with normal lungs, this presents no problems; however, for someone with lung disease, it is likely to mean that extra oxygen will be needed.

With the appropriate treatment, which is simply getting extra oxygen to breathe, it's remarkable how much better a person can feel. The various ways to obtain oxygen are outlined in *Appendix B: Medications*.

Respiratory Failure

As its name implies, respiratory failure is the condition where the job of the respiratory system is not being accomplished, which is usually defined by the blood oxygen level being too low, and the blood carbon dioxide level being too high. This problem can occur in different people for different reasons (see *Gas Transfer and Delivery*). Most often, respiratory failure occurs at least partly because of lung disease. If the lungs are very severely affected by CF, it may be difficult for oxygen to be absorbed into the bloodstream at the alveoli; there will also be airway obstruction which can be so great that the work of breathing becomes too difficult for the ventilatory muscles. Except in very rare cases, this does not happen suddenly in CF. When respiratory failure *does* occur in someone with CF, it is in someone who has had severe lung disease for a long time.

Treatment of respiratory failure

Respiratory failure is another complication of CF where the best treatment is simply a continuation and intensification of the usual treatments aimed at reducing bronchial obstruction, infection, and inflammation. In many cases, however, respiratory failure occurs only after the usual treatments have failed, and there is so little healthy lung tissue remaining that it cannot sustain the functions of bringing adequate amounts of oxygen into the body and eliminating enough carbon dioxide. If the oxygen level is low enough and/or the carbon dioxide level high enough, this is clearly a life-threatening situation. (You may want to refer back to *Anatomy and Function of the Respiratory System* to review why this is so serious.)

In desperation, physicians and families may consider using a mechanical ventilator to do the extra breathing for the patient. In some special circumstances, this may be effective, and may support the sick patient long enough for the lungs to improve, so that independent life is once again possible. These rare instances include respiratory failure that occurs suddenly and in a previously well patient, for example, as a result of an automobile accident or, rarely, as a result of a sudden serious viral infection like influenza. Respiratory failure in infants under the age of one year is also a special circumstance in which temporary support with a mechanical ventilator may be helpful.

However, in most cases where respiratory failure occurs, it is at the end of a long process, and the use of a mechanical ventilator does not reverse that process. The majority of patients with CF who are put on mechanical ventilators either die while still on the ventilator or are never able to come off it, despite weeks or even months of very intensive care. In order for a ventilator to work, a patient needs to have a tube in the trachea (either through the nose or mouth, or as a tracheotomy tube, through an incision in the neck). These tubes are uncomfortable, and make it impossible to talk. Ventilator support almost always means living in an intensive care unit, where there is usually little or no privacy, little differentiation between day and night, and constant monitoring by machines and people.

Heart–lung transplantation is a fairly new procedure in which a patient's lungs and heart are removed from the chest and a new set of lungs and heart put in their place. By 1988, this procedure had been performed in over 200 people with various kinds of lung problems. Fewer than three dozen patients with CF have received heart–lung transplants, and many have died. A few patients have done well, though, and have been able to go back to work and resume a reasonably active life. As with any new procedure, results are poor at first and improve as more experience is gained with them. At the time of the writing of this book, most experts consider heart–lung transplantation to be experimental for patients with CF. As time goes on, it may be that the techniques will have improved enough that the procedure will offer hope for some people with CF. A particular difficulty with this procedure is that one's chances of survival are related to how healthy one is at the time of the transplant. If one is so ill that death would be certain without the transplant, then the chances of surviving the operation as well as the post-operative medications and complications are relatively small. If one is healthy enough to withstand the operation and its consequences, then it is difficult to decide that one needs it.

Clearly, *the best treatment for respiratory failure is* **prevention**.

Cor Pulmonale and Heart Failure

Cor pulmonale literally means "heart disease caused by lung disease or breathing problems." Whenever the lungs are very severely affected (from almost any disease, including CF), or when the blood oxygen level is very low (from any cause), it becomes difficult for the heart to pump blood through the blood vessels in the lungs. Since it is the right side of the heart that pumps blood through the lungs, the right side of the heart gets a lot more exercise than usual. As with any other muscle, heart muscle will enlarge after it's had a lot of strenuous exercise. People who have had fairly severe lung disease for a period of time will commonly have a thick right-sided heart muscle, a condition called *right ventricular hypertrophy.* Not only will the muscle become thicker, but the whole right side of the heart may also expand. This enlargement is the way the heart adapts to the excess work it's being asked to do. It is most often a *successful* adaptation. Since this is a successful adjustment by the heart to a difficult situation, it is not considered heart disease. Though there is an abnormal *shape* and *size* to the right ventricle of the heart, this is quite different from disease, which is, by definition, harmful. Right ventricular hypertrophy is the *healthy* adjustment to the abnormally great demands placed on the normal heart by the diseased lungs.

If the lung disease remains too severe for too long, the heart may no longer be able to meet all the demands placed on it. It may not be able to pump all the blood that's necessary, and some fluid may back up. This fluid can sometimes be noticed in the ankles and lower legs, and sometimes a feeling of fullness in the right side of the abdomen under the ribs signifies fluid build-up in the liver. When the heart muscle fails to pump its entire assigned load, we say there is "heart failure," which is a frightening and misleading name for the condition, because it makes one think of heart *stoppage,* which it is not. Heart failure is the failure of the heart to do its *full* job. It is a serious problem, but one that indicates a serious lung problem rather than a problem with the heart itself.

Treatment of cor pulmonale and heart failure

Once again, the most effective treatment for this complication of CF lung disease is the aggressive treatment of the lung disease itself. In some cases, where there is excess fluid, a diuretic medication may be helpful (see *Appendix B: Medications*).

Chest pain

Chest pain is a fairly common complication of CF and has many different causes. The major cause is pneumothorax. This is usually a sharp pain, that occurs suddenly, is limited to one side, and is accompanied by shortness of breath. Other problems, while not as dangerous as pneumothorax, can be just as bothersome. The musculoskeletal system can be the source of chest pain in CF, especially when someone is coughing a lot: strained muscles, pulled tendons, bruised or even broken ribs can occur. Infection involving the pleura (the membrane surrounding the lung) can be very uncomfortable,

NORMAL

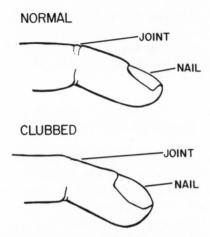

CLUBBED

FIG. 1.9. Digital (finger) clubbing. The clubbed finger is flattened at the angle where the nail meets the skin, and the tip of the finger is thicker than usual.

especially with deep breaths or coughs. This problem is called *pleuritis,* or sometimes *pleurisy.* Although anatomy books state that bronchi do not have pain-sensing nerves, some CF physicians think that pain may arise from large mucous plugs caught in small bronchi: clearly, some patients experience pain that disappears after they have coughed up a large plug of mucus. In younger people, the chest tightness that may accompany an asthma attack or a pulmonary exacerbation may seem like pain. Finally, there are nonpulmonary causes for chest pain in CF (heart attack is *not* among these): inflammation of the esophagus from acid reflux (see Chapter 2) can cause "heartburn," which may be accompanied by difficulty in swallowing; and psychologic stress can certainly cause chest pain.

Bone and Joint Problems

People with CF who have absolutely no lung problems will not have any skeletal problems that can be attributed to CF. However, almost everyone with CF who has even the slightest degree of lung involvement (and that means almost everyone with CF) will have a condition called *digital clubbing.* This is an unfortunate name for this condition, since it sounds rather grotesque, and while in its most extreme form it can be very noticeable, in most cases it affects only slightly the shape of the fingers and toes. As shown in Figure 1.9, two features distinguish clubbed fingers from nonclubbed fingers: the first is the angle at which the base of the nail meets the finger. This angle becomes progressively flatter as clubbing increases. The second characteristic of a clubbed finger is that the thickness of the tip of the finger, the part beyond the last joint, when measured from the base of the nail to the bottom of the finger pad, becomes thicker than the finger at the joint itself.

The cause of digital clubbing is not known. In general, as lung disease worsens, so does clubbing. However, many people with fairly mild lung disease may also have pronounced clubbing. Therefore, clubbing itself does not precisely reflect the degree of lung involvement.

There are other conditions aside from CF that are associated with clubbing, including some forms of liver disease, inflammatory bowel disease, and heart diseases in which the blood oxygen level is too low. Clubbing is a very helpful diagnostic clue when a child with lung problems is being evaluated, since clubbing is found in most CF patients over the age of 1 or 2 years, and is very rare in children who do not have CF. Any child with chronic or recurrent respiratory problems and digital clubbing should be tested for CF.

Another complication of CF which may affect the skeletal system is one that causes bone or joint pain in the legs, particularly the knees. This problem is called *hypertrophic pulmonary osteoarthropathy* (HPOA). The name indicates that it is seen in people with pulmonary problems, and refers to "something wrong with" (*-opathy*) the "bones" (*osteo*) and/or "joints" (*arthro*). The term *hypertrophic* refers to X-ray examination of the condition, which reveals that the periosteum, or membrane covering the bone, is usually elevated, appearing as though there is "extra" (*hyper*) "growth" (*trophy*). The condition can be painful. It is not very common, and occurs mostly in people whose lung disease is severe. It usually improves as the lungs improve with treatment, but specific treatment for the bone/joint problem can also be helpful.

Treating bone and joint problems

The degree of digital clubbing roughly corresponds with the degree of lung involvement, so treating the lungs may indirectly lessen the amount of clubbing. There is no treatment for clubbing aside from treatment of the lungs. Fortunately, a specific treatment is not required for clubbing, since it is not a painful condition. The only problem with clubbing is the embarrassment it can cause in adjusting to having fingers that look different from normal.

Osteoarthropathy may cause some physical discomfort, and people often will not mention it to their CF physicians, being unaware that leg or knee pain could be related to CF. As with clubbing, osteoarthropathy improves when the lungs improve. Regardless of the condition of the lungs, the discomfort of osteoarthropathy responds very well to aspirin, ibuprofen, and other similar antiinflammatory drugs (see *Appendix B: Medications*).

TESTS

Several kinds of tests can give important objective information about the lungs in someone with CF. These tests may be useful to confirm the physician's or patient's assessment of the patient's condition, to guide treatment, to measure the response to treatment, or in some cases to identify a problem before it has become evident to family or physician. Since most problems can be treated best if they are discovered early, many CF centers employ these tests on a regular basis, and not just when there is obvious trouble.

Pulmonary Function Tests

Pulmonary Function Tests (PFT's) are tests that measure various aspects of lung function. They can determine lung size, and presence and degree of bronchial obstruction. They can even give a good idea of which bronchi are blocked (the smallest bronchi or the larger central airways). They can identify asthma in children and adults, and they can measure the amount of oxygen circulating in the blood.

PFT's are a sensitive tool for following the condition of someone's lungs, showing subtle changes which might not have been detected otherwise. Since most PFT's require the understanding and cooperation of the patient, children under the age of 6 or 7 years may not be able to do these tests.

Spirometry

Spirometry ("measuring breathing") is the simplest PFT and is available in most hospitals and clinics. In this test, the patient breathes in and out through a tube while the machine records the amount of air breathed and the speed at which it is blown out.

Figure 1.10 shows two kinds of graphs that the spirometer can produce. The first (Figure 1.10a) records the amount (volume) of air blown out after the largest possible inhalation, and the time it takes to exhale it forcefully. Most of the air is exhaled in the first second, and all of it by 3 seconds. The most basic measurement from this curve is the *forced vital capacity* (FVC), the volume of air that is blown out in a single maximum exhaled breath. The next most commonly used measurement is the *forced expired volume in 1 second* (FEV_1), since this is a good indicator of whether there is blockage, and how much, particularly in the large central bronchi. The more obstruction there is, the more difficult it is to get air out of the lungs quickly, and the smaller the FEV_1. This is illustrated on the graph, where the solid line is from someone who has CF and normal lung function, and the dotted line is from someone who has CF and a moderate amount of obstruction.

The *maximum voluntary ventilation* (MVV) is similar to the spirometric tests just discussed. It calculates the maximum amount of air that someone can breathe in and out in 1 minute. The test doesn't last a whole minute, though. In most labs, the technician cheers and yells and vigorously encourages you to "Blow! Blow! Blow!" for either 12 or 15 seconds. The volume of air you've been able to breathe is then multiplied by 5 (for a 12-

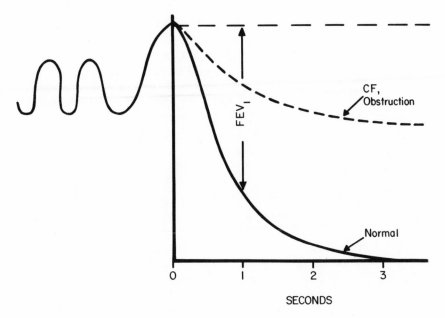

A

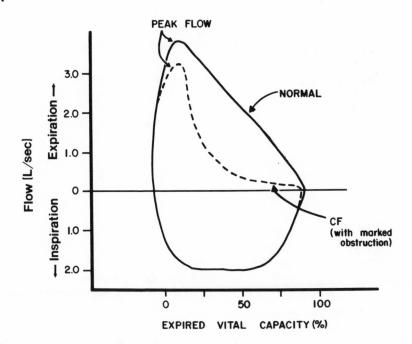

B

FIG. 1.10. Pulmonary function tests. **A**: Spirometry. **B**: Flow–volume curve. (See text for discussion.)

second test) or 4 (for a 15-second test) to give a value for 1 minute's worth of all out effort.

These tests (FVC, FEV_1, MVV) are useful, but they have one important drawback, namely, they are very "effort-dependent," meaning that a half-hearted breath will give worthless information. Experienced technicians can very often tell from the shape of the curve whether the patient has given as good an effort as possible. Newer machines may print out numbers for the FVC and FEV_1, rather than a curve. With these machines it is extremely difficult to evaluate the information, since it is difficult to determine how reliable the effort was that went into the breath.

Another way of looking at the information from spirometry is the *flow–volume curve* (Fig. 1.10b), which shows how quickly air flows out of the lungs at different points during a maximum expiratory effort. This gives valuable information because air comes out much faster at the beginning of a breath, when the lungs are fully inflated, than it does later on in the breath, when the lungs are nearly empty. The flow–volume curve relates the flow rates to precise portions of the breath. For example, the MEF_{25} is the maximum expiratory flow rate at 25 percent of vital capacity, meaning it is the rate at which air flows out of the lungs during a maximum effort at the point when exactly 75 percent of the breath is gone (and 25 percent remains in the lungs). Another reason this information is so useful is that the flow rates during the second half of a breath out depend very little on how hard a breath is taken; that is, these flow rates are relatively effort-independent, and are therefore valuable even in someone whose cooperation is less than perfect. Finally, the flow rates at the end of a breath seem to be a good reflection of the amount of obstruction in the smallest bronchi: during the first part of the exhalation, the air quickly empties out of the larger bronchi, and during the last half or quarter of the breath the air empties out of the smallest bronchi. Therefore, a slower than normal second half of a breath can indicate some blockage in the smallest airways, even when the larger bronchi are unobstructed and the first half of the breath is perfectly normal.

Lung Volumes

Lung volumes are measured by two different methods and require complex machinery, which may not be available in every physician's office or hospital. Yet they can give valuable information that cannot be obtained with spirometry. Spirometry measures the air that moves in and out of the lungs, but indicates nothing about the actual size of the lungs or the amount of air left inside the lungs after a person has finished blowing out.

The *helium dilution method* for measuring lung volumes uses the "Iced Tea Principle." If you place a teaspoon of sugar into a full glass of iced tea, and mix it thoroughly, the sweetness of the tea will depend on the size of the glass. Clearly, an 8-ounce glass will be much sweeter with a teaspoon of sugar than a quart jar. Another way of saying this is—the smaller the glass, the greater the concentration of sugar. In fact, if you had tools precise enough to measure the exact sweetness or the exact concentration of sugar, and you knew the exact amount of sugar you put in (1 teaspoon, in this case) you could calculate the size of the glass.

For measuring lung volumes, the sugar-substitute is helium, a gas that is very safe to breathe in and which is not absorbed into the bloodstream. If you breathe in a known amount of helium for a few minutes, until it is thoroughly mixed with the air in your lungs, the concentration of helium in the air you breathe out can tell the size of your lungs. This method works fairly well for determining the size of your lungs at their largest (with the biggest breath in), and at their smallest (after you've breathed out all you can). These are the *total lung capacity* and *residual volume,* respectively. The method is not perfect because it requires that all of the bronchial tubes be open so that the helium can mix completely with all areas of the lung. If a portion of one lung is blocked off, the helium won't mix with the air in that part of the lung, and it will seem that the lungs are smaller than they actually are. What is measured by this method is the volume of lung which freely communicates with the mouth; that's the same as the total lung volume if the airways are healthy, but in obstructed lungs the volume will be underestimated.

The "body box" (total body plethysmograph) solves the problem of obstruction. It is an expensive piece of equipment that looks something like a space capsule. Not many hospitals are equipped with body boxes suitable for testing children. The person being tested sits inside the box and breathes through a tube. When the box is shut, it is completely air-tight, which allows changes in pressure within the box to be measured very precisely while the person breathes. The changes in pressure reflect the changes in chest size. A mathematical formula is then applied that translates the pressure changes into accurate lung volume calculations, which include all of the lung volume, whether the bronchi are blocked or open. If someone does have bronchial obstruction, the total lung capacity will not be affected very much, but since obstruction (especially of small airways) makes it difficult to empty the lungs, the residual volume (the amount of air left in the lungs after a maximum exhalation) will be larger than normal. Normally, the residual volume is less than 25 percent of the total lung capacity, but in someone with severely blocked small airways, it can be as much as 70 percent of total lung capacity.

Asthma Testing

Asthma is a condition in which bronchi are blocked because of contraction of the muscles in the bronchial wall (this contraction of bronchial wall muscles is sometimes called *bronchospasm*). While the flow rates and lung volumes from the tests just described can tell if an obstruction is present, they can't tell what has caused it. However, if someone inhales a fast-acting bronchodilator, the bronchial muscle quickly relaxes, and the obstruction decreases. If the PFT's are repeated, the flow rates will show dramatic improvement within a few minutes. Since it's important to know how much obstruction is reversible, many labs will automatically schedule a bronchodilator inhalation and repeat spirometry as part of routine PFT's.

Some labs may go one step further, and try to identify people whose bronchi aren't yet blocked by bronchospasm but are *susceptible* to such blockage. These are people with **reactive airways**, which is another term for asthma. These people may have completely normal pulmonary function at a given time, but if they inhale certain chemicals, their bronchial muscles may contract much more readily than the bronchial muscles of someone with normal airways. To test for this, people may be asked to breathe in these chemicals (methacholine is the one most commonly used in this country; histamine is another), starting with a very dilute solution, and increasing step by step to a stronger solution, repeating the spirometry after each new challenge. The test is completed when the PFT's worsen. Someone has reactive airways disease if his or her PFT's get worse with a dilute (weak) solution of the chemical. These tests which measure airway reactivity are called *bronchial provocation* or *inhalation challenge tests*. Other bronchial challenge tests involve PFT's before and after exercise or before and after inhaling cold dry air.

Blood Gases

Since the major job of the lungs is to bring oxygen into the bloodstream and to eliminate carbon dioxide, it may be important to know the blood oxygen and carbon dioxide levels. To find this out, a blood gas test is performed by inserting a needle into an artery and drawing out blood. Since a needle inserted into an artery can be much more painful than one inserted into a vein, a small amount of xylocaine is injected into the skin first, which numbs the skin and makes the test tolerable.

Oximetry

Over the past few years, painless, noninvasive monitors have been developed which decrease the need for arterial blood gases. These monitors are called **oximeters** (either ear oximeters or pulseoximeters), and they work through a computerized method: a light is shined through the fingertip or earlobe to a sensor on the other side of the finger or ear; the amount of light that can pass through the tissues is determined partly by the amount of oxygen that is in the blood in those tissues. The oxygen saturation of the blood is calculated almost instantaneously by computer, and is indicated on a digital display.

Exercise Tests

Standard pulmonary function tests measure lung function while a person is resting. It may be useful in some situations to see how the lungs (and heart) function when they are put under some stress, as with exercise. Exercise tests can range from the very simple (listening to someone's lungs after he or she has been running in a hallway) to the very complex (measuring the precise amounts of oxygen consumed, carbon dioxide produced, oxygen exhaled, time it takes to inhale and exhale, rate of breathing, heart rate, etc.). Many physicians feel that the exercise test is more successful than regular PFT's in detecting mild problems. This is because a mild problem will not present itself unless the system is stressed, as when people exert themselves to the limit. For most exercise tests, the person being tested pedals on a stationary exercise cycle or walks/runs on a treadmill. The test begins with an easy pace, and gets increasingly difficult. While the test is going on, you may have to breathe through a mouthpiece like a scuba diver's, so that the air you breathe in and out can be analyzed. In other tests, you may have electrocardiogram (ECG) electrodes taped on your chest. In some tests, oximeters may be used, with a light taped to your finger or ear. In very special tests, there may even be a small plastic tube placed in the artery at your wrist. In other tests, none of those monitors may be used. Several laboratories are actively involved in research to determine the usefulness of routine exercise testing.

Chest X-rays

X-rays are generated by a machine that functions similarly to a camera. The X-ray machine is directed at the object to be studied, and generates X-rays, which pass through that object, in varying amounts and intensity. The X-rays then strike and expose photographic paper which is situated behind the object. When there is no object in the way, and the X-rays hit the photographic paper directly, it becomes completely black. When an object such as lead is in the way, which totally blocks all the X-rays, the paper becomes completely white. The thicker or more dense a material, the more rays it absorbs, and the whiter the image of that material on the resulting X-ray film. When the object in question is a person's chest, there will be recognizable white/black/gray patterns determined by the bones, lungs, heart, etc. The bones are quite dense, and therefore will appear white on the final X-ray. The heart, because it consists of thick muscle and is filled with blood, also appears fairly white. The lungs are much less dense, since they are

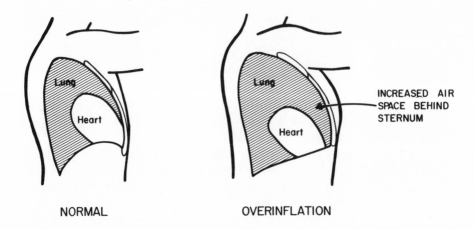

NORMAL   OVERINFLATION

FIG. 1.11. X-ray appearance of overinflation of lungs, with "bowing" of the sternum, and large collection of air behind sternum.

relatively delicate tissues largely filled with air, and therefore appear much blacker, or at least a darker shade of gray. The lungs do contain some dense tissue, including blood vessels, so they are not totally black. The diaphragms mark the lower edges of the lungs, and are white since they are fairly solid muscle.

Chest X-rays can give important information about the condition of the lungs. If, for example, a lobe of the lung is collapsed because it is filled with mucus, that lobe will appear much denser (whiter) than normal. If thick scar tissue has replaced healthy lung tissue, that too will be whiter than usual. Bronchial walls swollen by fluid or inflammation may have a similar appearance. In many cases it is possible to see "increased markings," meaning more white (dense) markings than normal, but it is not possible to tell if the increased density is caused by inflammation or mucus (which can get better), or by scar tissue (which cannot get better).

A pneumothorax, in which air has escaped through a leak in the lung but is still within the chest, will show up on the X-ray as a totally black area outside the lung, while the lung itself will be whiter than normal (see Fig. 1.6). The totally black area is air, and the lung will appear denser (whiter) than normal since it is partly collapsed, with the solid parts of the lung closer together than normal.

Lungs that are obstructed and difficult to empty will be larger than normal, and will push the diaphragms downward (Fig. 1.11). These overinflated (*hyperinflated*) lungs may not only push the diaphragms down into a flattened shape (compared with the normal dome shape), but may actually push the sternum (the front of the chest) forward. This is called *sternal bowing* (since the shape of the sternum comes to resemble an archery bow).

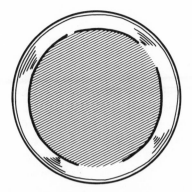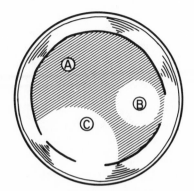

FIG. 1.12. Culture and sensitivity testing, showing clear zones around the antibiotic discs. The larger the clear space around the disc, the more potent the antibiotic has been in preventing the bacteria from growing.

Cultures and Sensitivities

It is important to know what bacteria are in the bronchi of someone with CF, in case antibiotic treatment becomes necessary. To identify bacteria, small samples of mucus are sent to a bacteriology laboratory where they are placed in different substances called *media*. Some media are good environments for all types of bacteria to grow in, and others will allow only certain bacteria to grow. After the bacteria have grown they are analyzed and identified, with the entire process taking several days.

Once the bacteria are grown and identified, the task remains of determining which antibiotics are the most effective in killing those bacteria. To find this out, various antibiotics are added to the cultures and their effects are observed. One method of introducing antibiotics is through the use of paper discs that have been soaked with the antibiotic. These discs are placed at intervals around the plate where the bacteria are grown (Fig. 1.12). If the antibiotic kills the bacteria, there will be a clear area around the disc, where the bacteria have not been able to grow (this clear area is called the *zone of inhibition*). If the bacteria are not killed by the antibiotic, they continue to grow right up to the disc, leaving no clear zone. Sometimes there will be a very small zone, sometimes a larger one. Most laboratories will define the response to the antibiotic based on the size of the clear zone. For example, when the antibiotic gentamicin is used in cultures of *Pseudomonas,* the bacteria are proclaimed *sensitive* to the antibiotic if the clear area is 15 mm or larger; if the clear area is 13–14 mm, it is considered *intermediate,* and if it is 12 mm or less, the bacteria are said to be *resistant* to the effects of the antibiotic. "Resistance" is thus a relative term, since the presence of even a very small clear space indicates that some bacteria have been killed.

SUMMARY

The respiratory system accounts for over 95 percent of the illness and deaths from CF, and therefore keeping it healthy is the most important thing that can be done for anyone with CF. Fortunately, there is much that can be done towards this end, and the tremendous improvement in life expectancy of CF patients can be attributed largely to better prevention and treatment of lung problems. Most of the problems that develop in the lung are the result of bronchial blockage caused by thick mucus, and of infection which follows the blockage. Physical means, such as postural drainage and percussion treatments, and medications including bronchodilators, help prevent and reverse bronchial obstruction. Antibiotics, given by mouth, aerosol, or injection, are very successful in treating bronchial infection.

2 / The Gastrointestinal Tract

Susan R. Orenstein and David M. Orenstein

THE NORMAL GASTROINTESTINAL TRACT

The gastrointestinal tract is made up of the organs that digest food (Fig. 2.1). One way to understand how the gastrointestinal tract normally works in people without cystic fibrosis (CF) is to think about what happens to the parts of a meal when they are eaten. For this purpose we can use a (not completely well-rounded) meal consisting of meat, potato with butter, a glass of whole milk, and a dessert of candy. Each of these foods has a mix of nutrients: *protein, fat,* and *carbohydrate.* For this discussion, however, the meat will represent its main component, protein; the potato, starch (a carbohydrate with complex branching chains of molecules); the butter, fat; and the candy, sucrose (a carbohydrate that is simpler than starch). The milk contains another simple carbohydrate, lactose, as well as fat and protein.

None of this food would stay in the body if it were not broken down into small particles that can be absorbed into the bloodstream. This breaking down process is called *digestion.* When a person eats such a meal, digestion begins immediately in the **mouth**. Saliva contains digestive enzymes called *amylase* and *lipase,* and when these are mixed with the food during chewing, the amylase starts to break down the starch of the potato and the lipase starts to break down the fat of the butter and milk. You will notice that most of the enzymes that break down food end in "-ase" or "-sin."

The **esophagus** is not actively involved in the process of digestion. It is a tube that moves the chewed food from the mouth to the stomach. It does have an important role, however, for it must move food down without air getting in, and it must let air or food come up when the need arises to belch or vomit. It is the esophagus that keeps food and liquid in the stomach, even when a person is upside down.

The chewed-up meat, potato, butter, milk, and candy have now passed through the esophagus into the **stomach**. Here, the protein in the meat and milk is acted upon by the enzyme *pepsin,* which is secreted by the stomach.

When the food has been ground up by the stomach into small particles,

51

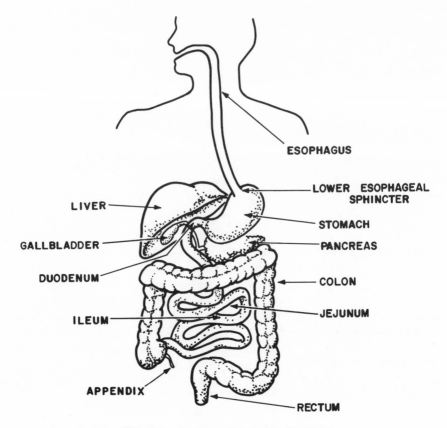

FIG. 2.1. Anatomy of gastrointestinal tract.

the partly digested food is released slowly into the **duodenum**, the first part of the **small intestine**. Several inches beyond the stomach, in the duodenum, is a tiny opening through which juices from the **liver** and **pancreas** flow into the duodenum. These juices contain large amounts of important digestive enzymes that are made by the pancreas, and bile salts (also called bile acids), which are made by the liver. Among the pancreatic enzymes are peptidases, which digest proteins. *Trypsin* and *chymotrypsin* are two protein-digesting enzymes that continue the digestion of the protein from the meat and milk after it has passed from the stomach. Two other important pancreatic enzymes are *amylase,* which like salivary amylase, continues to break down the potato's starch, and *lipase,* which digests nearly all the fat in the butter and milk. Lipase is a particularly important enzyme because it is the major fat-digesting enzyme in the digestive tract, and also because it is very fragile, and is destroyed when in the presence of too much acid. Lipase also has other requirements to function well—bile salts, made by the liver, and colipase, made by the pancreas, are both needed in the duodenum for lipase to work well.

The products of all of this digestion of protein and fat and starch are absorbed by the tiny cells of the wall of the small intestine as the muscles of the intestine squeeze the food slowly along toward the **large intestine** (also called the **colon**). There are enzymes attached to the cells of the wall of the small intestine that break down simple carbohydrates such as the sucrose of the candy and the lactose of the milk, just before they are absorbed by the intestinal cells. Other enzymes on these cells complete the digestion of starch and protein that was begun by the enzymes from the pancreas. Once the food has been broken down into these tiny particles and taken into the intestinal cells, it passes into the bloodstream and is carried to the various parts of the body where it is needed.

In a person whose gastrointestinal tract is working properly, nearly all of the nutritious food that is eaten is digested by the pancreatic enzymes and absorbed by the intestinal cells into the bloodstream. Very little of the food gets to the colon. That person's bowel movements contain indigestible fiber from the food, some water to keep the movement soft, and quite a lot of the bacteria that normally live in the large intestine. Very little of the carbohydrate and protein, and less than 7 percent of the fat, is wasted.

THE GASTROINTESTINAL TRACT IN CYSTIC FIBROSIS

The remainder of this chapter is devoted to the problems that occur in the gastrointestinal tract in patients with CF, with each problem being reviewed under the affected organ. Table 2.1 lists the problems and the frequency with which they occur.

Pancreas

Pancreatic Insufficiency

Abnormal mucus blocks the tiny tubes in the pancreas of people with CF, much as it does in the lungs. This means that the digestive enzymes are not secreted into the intestine as they should be. (Remember that these enzymes are *lipase,* which digests fat; *amylase,* which digests starch; and the *peptidases,* including trypsin and chymotrypsin and others, which digest proteins.) Pancreatic insufficiency refers to the inability of the pancreas to secrete *enough* digestive enzymes for normal digestion. This does not happen until nearly all (90 percent) of the normal enzyme activity is lost, so the pancreatic secretion must be quite low for pancreatic insufficiency to occur. Most infants with CF have pancreatic insufficiency, and the number of CF children with pancreatic insufficiency increases with age, so that 85–90 percent of all people with CF require treatment for pancreatic insufficiency.

TABLE 2.1. *Incidence of gastrointestinal tract conditions in cystic fibrosis*

Organ	Condition	% of CF patients with condition
Pancreas	Pancreatic insufficiency	85–90
	Pancreatitis	1
	Diabetes	1–5[a]
Liver and gallbladder	Cirrhosis	1–4
	Gallstones	10
Esophagus and stomach	Gastroesophageal reflux	10–20
	Ulcers	1–10
Intestines	Meconium ileus	10
	Meconium peritonitis	1
	Meconium ileus equivalent	10–30
	Rectal prolapse	10–20
	Intussusception	1

[a]Diabetes is extremely uncommon before the age of 10 years; thereafter, it occurs in about 10 percent of patients until age 20 years, and in another 10 percent from 20–30 years.

Before effective treatment was available, most CF children died in infancy, in part from starvation (malnutrition) due to their pancreatic insufficiency.

The intestinal cells have a "backup" group of enzymes that do fairly well at digesting starch and protein when the pancreas is not working properly. In this case, however, the digestion of starch is not complete, which may cause gas when it gets to the large intestine (colon). The digestion of protein is also not complete, so that some patients, especially infants, may have low levels of protein in the blood. If protein levels are sufficiently low, fluid may leak out of the blood vessels and cause puffy skin (edema).

The intestinal cells do not have a backup means to digest fat, and the effectiveness of the lipase produced by the salivary glands is limited. Therefore, most CF patients do not digest and absorb fat well, and fat is passed out of the body in the bowel movements. Fat makes the bowel movements large, greasy, and more smelly than normal. All of the fat that comes out in the bowel movements is lost to the body. A given amount of fat has more calories than any other kind of food, so losing an ounce of fat means losing more than twice as many calories as would be lost in an ounce of carbohydrate or protein. Loss of fat in the bowel movements thus leads to malnutrition and poor growth, despite an oftentimes huge appetite. Fat malabsorption may also lead to the lack of special kinds of fatty nutrients that are essential to health—"essential fatty acids," and fat-soluble vitamins (vitamins A, D, E, and K). (Vitamins are discussed more fully in Chapter 4.)

There are several ways in which a physician can determine if someone has pancreatic insufficiency. The first is simply a review of the history of bowel movements: frequent, greasy, smelly, large bowel movements usually indicate pancreatic insufficiency. A second method is a test that involves taking a small sample of stool (bowel movement), staining it with a dye that will make the fat present in the stool an easily noticeable color, and then examining it under the microscope. A large amount of fat indicates that fat was not digested and absorbed, and therefore suggests pancreatic insufficiency. Stool can also be analyzed for the amount of trypsin and chymotrypsin. Absent enzymes, or very low levels of enzymes, suggests that the pancreas has not released the enzymes. However, this test can be misleading, since some of the bacteria that live in the intestines can produce trypsin, while others can destroy it.

A more reliable test is the "Chymex test." In this test, the patient takes in a chemical by mouth. This chemical is composed of two ingredients, one of which is called PABA. When PABA and its partner stay together, they form a chemical that is so large that it passes through the body in the stools without being absorbed. But if PABA is separated from the other part of the chemical, the PABA can be absorbed and then passed out in the urine. Pancreatic chymotrypsin is the only substance that can separate PABA from its partner. Therefore, if PABA appears in the urine, then chymotrypsin must have been available from the pancreas.

A final test for pancreatic insufficiency is much more invasive than those just discussed. This test involves passing a tube through the nose, esophagus, and stomach into the duodenum, then collecting fluid directly from the point at which the pancreas empties its enzymes. The fluid can then be analyzed directly for enzyme content.

One further test that is being used primarily as a newborn screening test for CF also relates to pancreatic function. This is a blood test which is performed on the first or second day of life. A dried spot of blood is analyzed for immunoreactive trypsin (IRT), a substance that is found in higher quantities in the blood of newborns with CF than in those without CF. It is not known why this is so, but it may be that the trypsin, which can't get out of the pancreas into the duodenum, "backs up" into the bloodstream. One problem with this explanation is that the 10 percent of CF babies who don't have pancreatic insufficiency may have an abnormal IRT. The test is hardly perfect for identifying CF, since there are many *false positives* (babies who don't have CF, but who test abnormal for IRT). Nevertheless, the test may have some value, and its use is being examined in the United States and in several countries around the world.

Treatment of pancreatic insufficiency is fairly simple and the results are dramatic, now that pancreatic enzyme replacement is possible through the use of granules, powder, or capsules taken with meals. These enzymes are often *enteric coated*, meaning that they are protected from the stomach acid by a coating that dissolves only when it is in a nonacidic surrounding. These enzymes pass through the stomach and begin to dissolve in the duodenum, which is a nonacidic environment (see *Appendix B: Medications*). The quantity of enzymes to be taken is determined by evaluating such factors as weight gain and bowel movements.

The amount of enzyme taken must be adjusted properly, since too much enzyme can cause problems (rarely, children may become constipated from high quantities of enzyme). Since the CF pancreas also does not produce acid-neutralizing juice as does the normal pancreas, the duodenum may be fairly acidic, and enteric-coated enzymes may not be properly activated. Therefore, some CF children need treatment with antacids, cimetidine, or ranitidine to make their enzymes work. Infants who are given the enzymes as nonenteric-coated granules or powder may develop an irritation around mouth or bottom, and mothers who are breast-feeding these infants may develop nipple irritation. For these reasons, the enteric-coated enzymes are usually much better than nonenteric-coated, especially in infants. (See *Appendix B: Medications,* for more details about taking enzymes.)

Pancreatitis

Pancreatitis is an inflammation of the pancreas that causes severe abdominal pain and usually vomiting. It occurs in people without CF, sometimes due to gallstones blocking the pancreas' secretion, sometimes due to drinking alcohol, sometimes as a side effect of medications, and sometimes for unknown reasons. Adolescents, adults, or older children with CF who do *not* have pancreatic insufficiency may get pancreatitis, but this is quite rare. Pancreatitis is diagnosed with blood and urine tests and with X-rays. It is treated with a stay in the hospital, during which no food is given by mouth and nutrition is given intravenously. Taking pancreatic enzymes may also help this problem to resolve.

Diabetes

In addition to producing digestive enzymes and juices, the pancreas produces hormones, especially insulin. Insulin is needed by the body to put glucose, the body's main simple carbohydrate used for energy, into cells. When insulin is not produced as it is needed, blood glucose (*blood sugar*) rises, and diabetes results.

Diabetes involves many complicated processes in the body. The high blood glucose causes glucose to be lost in the urine, and this glucose takes water with it that is needed by the body. The loss of glucose and water from the body produces other changes that can make people with diabetes malnourished, dehydrated, and quite ill.

Nearly one-half of all people with CF have some limitation of the ability of their pancreas to produce insulin, which is detectable with special tests. However, only a very small proportion of CF patients have diabetes—that is, glucose lost in their urine. Almost no one under the age of 10 years has this problem, and between the ages of 10 and 20 years, approximately 10 percent of CF patients develop it. From the ages of 20–30 years, another 10 percent develop it, and so forth, with an additional 10 percent developing diabetes with every additional decade. The diabetes in CF patients tends to be milder than the diabetes in other children, and is less apt to produce serious illness. The treatment for diabetes involves taking insulin by injection every day.

Intestines

Meconium Ileus

Meconium is a baby's first bowel movement, formed in the intestine while the baby is still in the mother's womb. Since the baby has had nothing to eat, this bowel movement is formed from bits of mucus and intestinal cells shed into the intestines before birth. It is usually darker and stickier than the infant's stools will be once he or she starts taking milk.

In infants with CF, the meconium is much thicker and stickier than usual, probably because of the abnormal sticky mucus that CF patients seem to make throughout the body. In a fair number of babies with CF (about 10 percent), this meconium is so thick that it clogs in the ileum [the third part of the small intestine, right near the appendix (see Fig. 2.1)] and blocks up the intestines. This condition is called *meconium ileus*. This prevents the baby from having a bowel movement, and also causes the abdomen to swell—usually within the first 2 days after birth. In such babies, meconium ileus is often the first clue that they have CF. Sometimes the intestines get so filled because of the blockage that a hole is broken in the intestinal wall, and meconium escapes into the abdomen. This is called *meconium peritonitis,* and can make the baby quite sick. It occurs in about 10 percent of infants with meconium ileus, which is approximately 1 percent of all infants with CF.

Treatment for meconium ileus can be given with special X-rays and enemas, but sometimes surgery is required. The X-ray and enema, called a *Gastrografin enema,* involves putting Gastrografin into the rectum, and letting it run back through the colon. Gastrografin is a liquid with three characteristics that make it ideal to use in this situation: (1) it is very slippery and can get by just about any obstruction; (2) it is very concentrated and acts like a dry sponge, pulling fluid into the intestines and watering down the thick meconium; and (3) it appears on an X-ray, so the progress of the whole procedure can be followed. When this procedure is carried out by radiologists experienced in its use in infants (ideally with the cooperation of surgeons and CF specialists), it is safe and very effective. However, in some infants, these enemas will not relieve the obstruction and surgery becomes necessary. All infants with meconium peritonitis require surgery. When the sur-

gery is performed by surgeons with experience in infants, it is usually successful. Babies who have had surgery have a slightly higher likelihood of
developing intestinal obstruction later in life because after abdominal surgery in *anyone* (infants or older people; CF or non-CF), scars (adhesions)
may form and block the intestines.

Meconium ileus is a serious problem, but most infants who have it do very
well after it is treated. If they make it through the difficult first few weeks,
their outlook is similar to other CF babies who have not had meconium ileus.
Meconium ileus occurs only in infants with CF; therefore, a baby with meconium ileus should be diagnosed immediately and general CF care should
begin right away.

Meconium Ileus Equivalent (Distal Intestinal Obstruction Syndrome)

This problem involves blockage of the intestines that is similar to meconium ileus, but occurs after infancy. The intestinal contents usually block the
same area of the ileum (just before the colon) as in meconium ileus, but
sometimes the blockage occurs farther along, in the colon. The term meconium ileus equivalent is used, even though intestinal contents are not referred
to as "meconium" in anyone older than a newborn.

Meconium ileus equivalent may be brought on by too few enzymes (since
that will make the stools very large and bulky), or by dietary changes, and
it is somewhat more common in children who have had meconium ileus as
newborns, especially if they had surgery. In rare cases, it may be caused by
an excess of enzymes. In many cases, it is not known what caused the blockage, other than the thickening of the intestinal mucus.

Crampy stomach aches and constipation are the symptoms produced by
meconium ileus equivalent, and often the blockage can be felt by the doctor
or seen on X-rays. If a person with CF has severe abdominal pain and no
bowel movements, it is most likely due to this problem.

Treatment for this complication of CF may involve continuing enzymes,
taking stool softeners or special laxative preparations, and having special X-
ray and enemas. Although it rarely requires surgery, it must be attended to
promptly so that more serious problems, such as bursting or leaking of the
bowels, do not occur.

Intussusception

Intussusception is a very rare problem which occurs when part of the intestine folds in on itself, and is pulled along inside the intestine in much the
same way that a telescope collapses in on itself (Fig. 2.2). Intussusception
can be a complication of meconium ileus equivalent, and the part of the
intestine that is pulled along is usually the end of the ileum, which is pulled

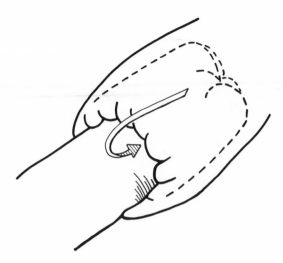

FIG. 2.2. Intussusception. This condition occurs when the intestine collapses within itself.

into the colon. What probably causes this action is that sticky stool and mucus, which adhere to the inside of the intestines, are pulled along by the powerful waves that pull the food along, drawing the intestine with them. This "telescoping" may cause the blood vessels that normally nourish the intestines to be blocked off, which may damage the intestine, causing bleeding or even destruction of that part of the bowel. Intussusception, like meconium ileus equivalent, causes abdominal pain (which may be intermittent or constant), and may cause vomiting or a decreased number of bowel movements. Intussusception may be treated by barium enema X-ray, or may require surgery, but patients with this problem tend to do well if promptly treated.

Rectum

Rectal Prolapse

Rectal prolapse is similar to intussusception, involving the same "telescoping" action. In this case, the rectum is pulled along through, and right out, of the anus, to a point that it becomes visible (Fig. 2.3). This usually happens during a bowel movement. Rectal prolapse often occurs repeatedly in a young child, before the diagnosis of CF is made. It is fairly common, occurring in nearly 20 percent of patients with CF. Though it is frightening for a parent to see, it is seldom dangerous or painful.

Rectal prolapse may be the first CF-related problem to appear before a child is diagnosed with CF. Several factors related to undiagnosed CF can

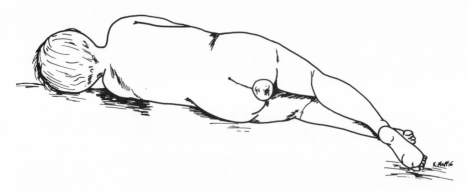

FIG. 2.3. Rectal prolapse. This condition is similar to intussusception in that the bowel turns partly inside-out. In rectal prolapse, the last part of the bowel, the rectum, turns inside-out and protrudes from the anus.

cause rectal prolapse. Malnutrition affects the structures that usually support the rectum, and coughing and straining during sticky, bulky bowel movements increases the pressure on the rectum, pushing it out. Treatment of each episode of prolapse usually consists simply of pushing the rectum gently back into place by hand. If it is difficult to restore it to its normal position, then a doctor's help should be obtained immediately. The prolapse usually stops occurring when treatment of the CF (especially with enzymes) improves the bowel movements, coughing decreases, and overall nutrition improves. Rectal prolapse rarely requires surgery. Since rectal prolapse is very uncommon in developed countries except in youngsters with CF, anyone with rectal prolapse should be tested for CF.

Esophagus

Gastroesophageal Reflux

Gastroesophageal reflux occurs when the stomach contents (consisting of acid made by the stomach and partially digested food) come back up into the esophagus. A certain amount of this is normal, and we are usually unaware that it is happening. However, when this occurs often, or when the acid from the stomach remains in the esophagus for very long, the mucous membranes of the esophagus become irritated and inflamed. *Esophagitis* (inflammation of the esophagus) then results, producing the feeling called "heartburn," which has nothing to do with the heart. In addition to the discomfort this causes, on rare occasions the damage can be severe enough to cause scarring of the esophagus (stricture) or bleeding.

Gastroesophageal reflux can lead to other problems in addition to the irritation of the esophagus itself. One problem occurs when the refluxed material comes up farther than the esophagus, and is actually vomited. Besides being messy, vomiting entails a loss of food and crucial nutrients which, if occurring frequently, can lead to malnutrition. This is a particular problem in babies who have reflux, because a baby's esophagus is much shorter than that of older children. Although a certain amount of "spitting up" is quite normal in babies, too much may be harmful, such as when it causes poor weight gain.

In addition to the irritation of the esophagus and the loss of calories, gastroesophageal reflux can cause pulmonary (lung or breathing) problems. This may occur two different ways: (1) refluxed material may reach the back of the throat and actually be breathed (aspirated) into the lungs. There are normally quite good protections that keep refluxed material from getting into the lungs, so most breathing problems caused by reflux occur in the second way; (2) when nerves in the esophagus are irritated by stomach acid, they can send a signal to the bronchial tubes in the lungs to get narrower, making the bronchi squeeze down. [In certain instances, this reaction is actually a protective mechanism (see Chapter 1, *Anatomy and Function of the Respiratory System*).] This reaction of the bronchi causes breathing difficulties that are similar to those of asthma, and may make the breathing problems of CF worse.

Several factors are responsible for the occurrence of reflux in people with CF. Some medications and treatments have a side effect of relaxing the muscle at the bottom of the esophagus (lower esophageal sphincter) (see Fig. 2.1). If that sphincter relaxes too much, food is more likely to pass through it into the esophagus. People with CF spend more time upside down (for treatments) than other people. If the muscle at the bottom of the esophagus relaxes when you are upright, gas escapes and we call that a burp, but if it happens when you are upside down, the stomach contents escape into the esophagus. Coughing, which is helpful in clearing lung mucus, also tightens the abdominal muscles, and may put pressure on the stomach that forces material up into the esophagus. People with CF may produce more stomach acid than normal, and this may also make reflux worse.

Treatment for reflux is divided into three categories: simple measures, medications, and surgery. The simple measures include position and meal characteristics. Head-down positions and lying on the back or slouching while sitting make reflux worse. Infant seats, which put babies in a partly back-lying and partly slouching position, can cause infants to have more reflux than when they are lying face down. Sitting or standing straight up, and lying face down, make reflux less likely to occur. Elevating the head of the bed 6–12 inches by raising the bed legs on blocks will also help. Meals should be eaten at least two hours before bed, and acid foods (tomatoes, soft drinks, juices) should be avoided. Thickening infants' formula with 1 tablespoon of dry rice cereal for each ounce of formula helps decrease spitting up, and also adds calories to the formula. Smoking (or being around smoke) and caffeine may also make reflux worse, so children with CF and reflux should avoid exposure to these things. (Of course, the smoke has an even worse effect on the lungs themselves, so there are several reasons to avoid being around smoke.)

Medications used to treat reflux include bethanechol (Urecholine) and metoclopramide (Reglan) (see *Appendix B: Medications*), which strengthen the muscle at the bottom of the esophagus. Since bethanechol may add to lung problems, and since metoclopramide may be of more benefit by also causing the stomach to empty into the intestine faster, metoclopramide is probably the better of the two. Its main side effect, when the dose is too high for a patient, is a restlessness, which may progress to back-arching and stiffening, with eyes rolling back. This very rare side effect looks frightening, but is easily treated by stopping the medication and by receiving an injection of diphenhydramine (Benadryl) from a physician. Other medications that may be used to treat reflux include cimetidine and ranitidine, which decrease the stomach's production of acid, and liquid antacids, which neutralize the acid that has been produced.

If the simple measures and medications do not produce enough relief from the reflux, a surgical procedure called a *fundoplication* (or a Nissen fundoplication) can be performed. This involves wrapping the upper part of the stomach around the bottom of the esophagus to strengthen the muscle at the bottom of the esophagus. When performed by a surgeon experienced in children's problems, this is nearly always successful in treating reflux.

Stomach

Increased Acid

There may be an increase in the amount of acid the stomach makes in CF. Though this does not seem to make ulcers common in people with CF, it may add to the problem of gastroesophageal reflux and cause pancreatic enzymes to be less effective. These possibilities have been discussed in other sections.

Liver

Fatty Liver

The livers of people with CF fairly often become enlarged because the liver cells get packed with fat. This also happens in malnourished people without CF and it may be due to the malnutrition itself. (It is not known why malnutrition, which makes the rest of the body lose fat, makes the liver gain fat.) Fatty liver may happen at any age, and may improve as nutrition improves. It does not by itself cause any problems.

Blocked Bile Ducts

In addition to blocking the small tubes in the lungs and in the pancreas, abnormal sticky mucus can block the bile ducts. The bile ducts are the small tubes in the liver that take the bile, including the bile salts needed for digestion, to the pancreatic duct and then to the duodenum. Thus, when the bile ducts become blocked, it may increase the difficulties of fat digestion, since fat digestion requires that bile salts reach the intestine.

When the bile ducts become blocked in babies, the yellow bile cannot get out of the liver and backs up into the blood, where it is carried to the skin, causing a temporary yellow discoloration of the skin called *jaundice*. Jaundice in CF infants is much more common in those who have meconium ileus, the blockage of the intestines which has already been discussed. In older children, the blocked ducts are less likely to cause jaundice, but they may cause scarring in the liver (biliary fibrosis), which may often be present without producing any signs or problems. If this scarring becomes severe, it is called *biliary cirrhosis* and can cause serious problems. This may happen in a CF patient during the teenage years or later, but is quite rare, occurring in only 1–4 percent of people with CF.

The complex problems caused by cirrhosis of the liver include fluid (ascites) building up in the abdomen, and life-threatening bleeding from large veins (varices) that form in the esophagus. A third problem resulting from cirrhosis is called *hypersplenism*: The spleen, an organ in the left side of the abdomen, swells up and traps blood cells flowing through it. If it traps blood-clotting cells called platelets, it may cause bleeding problems; if it traps the red blood cells, there may be anemia.

If cirrhosis becomes severe enough, it may cause the liver to fail to work at all. Since the liver is essential to life, this is a cause of death in a small percentage (1–2 percent) of CF patients.

There is no known way at present to interrupt the scarring caused by the duct blockage in the liver, any more than in the pancreas. However, there are treatments for some of the problems caused by the liver scarring. Bile salts are part of some enzyme preparations used for people with CF, such as Accelerase and Cotazym-B, although neither of these is enteric-coated (see Chapter 4), and the enteric coating seems to be more important to the function of the enzymes than are the bile salts. If hypersplenism causes dangerously low levels of a particular type of blood cells, they can be replenished by transfusion, but this is rarely needed. If varices form and bleed, they can be treated by a procedure called *sclerotherapy*. This is a procedure in which a flexible, lighted tube is passed down the throat, and a material is injected into these large vessels in order to scar them closed. Sclerotherapy is usually repeated at intervals ranging from weeks to many months, and is quite effective in treating varices.

Another method used to treat varices is a surgical operation that directs the blood flow away from the varices; this is called a *shunt* or *porto-systemic shunt*.

Ascites, the collection of fluid in the abdomen, can be treated by changes in the amount of salt and water a person eats, and by drugs (diuretics) that increase urination. There are other treatments for the complexities of liver failure, which your doctor can discuss with you if they are ever needed.

Gallbladder

The gallbladder is a pouch attached to the bile ducts just outside the liver. It collects the bile made by the liver, and releases it into the intestine at the time of a meal, when it is needed. The gallbladder and the tube that connects it to the liver are abnormal in one-third of the people with CF, but this does not usually cause any problems. Approximately 10 percent of all CF patients may have gallstones. If they cause pain, which they sometimes do, they are treated by surgery to remove the gallbladder and the stones.

Abdominal Pain

"Stomach aches" are a common problem for people with CF, and there are many possible causes. Several of the complications listed in Table 2.1 cause abdominal pain. Meconium ileus equivalent may be the most common cause of stomach aches, but gallstones, ulcers, pancreatitis (only in those patients who do not require extra enzymes), and intussusception all of which occur more often in CF patients than in other people, are also major causes of abdominal problems. For patients who take enzyme supplements, it is important to take them regularly, for skipping enzymes is almost guaranteed to result in discomfort. Other sources of abdominal pain include excessive coughing, which can cause the abdominal muscles to become sore, and medications, some of which cause abdominal pain as well. People with CF can have the same abdominal problems as everyone else, including constipation, gastroenteritis (this is an intestinal infection, often inaccurately called a "stomach flu," and is frequently accompanied by nausea, vomiting, and/or diarrhea), urinary tract infection, and appendicitis. Ten percent of all white people have pain because of intolerance to lactose, the main carbohydrate in milk. In young women, gynecologic problems can be responsible for abdominal pain. Finally, psychologic stress can be a cause of stomach problems in some people.

3// Other Systems

David M. Orenstein

SWEAT GLANDS

Normal Sweat Glands

Sweat begins as a fluid that is chemically very similar to blood in the coil of the sweat gland, below the surface of the skin (Fig. 3.1). As it makes its way toward the skin, sodium—with its positive electrical charge—is pumped out of the duct, and eventually back to the bloodstream. Whenever a positive charge leaves any tube or duct in the body, a negative charge accompanies it in order to maintain the same total electrical charge. In the case of the sweat, it is chloride and its negative charge that are carried out of the sweat fluid to follow the positive charge of sodium. By the time the fluid reaches the skin surface in the form of sweat, it still has some salt, but the sodium and chloride contents are very low compared with that in the blood. This helps the body conserve sodium and chloride, especially in hot weather or when someone is exercising heavily.

Sweat Glands in Cystic Fibrosis

It has been known for many years that people with cystic fibrosis (CF) have an extremely high salt content in their sweat. In CF, the fluid passes up through the sweat duct system, and sodium is pumped out normally. Chloride, however, is somehow prevented from following the sodium out of the tube. It is not yet known why the mucous membrane of the sweat duct does not allow chloride to pass through it. The answer to this puzzle is sufficiently important that many scientists believe it may explain the basic defect underlying all the problems resulting from CF. It has already been discovered that the same chloride block occurs in the other organs affected by CF (pancreas, bronchi). (This is discussed more fully in Chapter 12.)

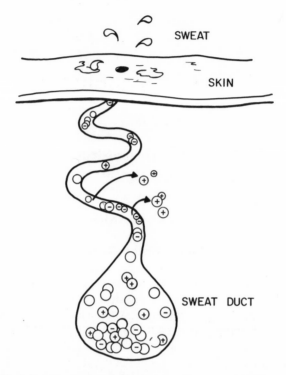

FIG. 3.1. Sweat abnormality. At the base of the sweat duct, both positive (sodium) and negative (chloride) charges are contained within the fluid. As the fluid moves upward toward the skin, the sodium with its positive charges are pumped out of the duct. The chloride with its negative charges are blocked from following, leaving many more negative (chloride) charges within the fluid as it reaches the skin as sweat.

The sweat abnormality is important for two reasons: (1) It allows the diagnosis of CF to be made through the sweat test, and (2) it means that some patients, especially babies, may become sick by losing more salt than they take in during the summer (see below: *Salt Loss*).

Over 99 percent of people with CF have abnormal sweat. They sweat the same amount of sweat, but there is an excess of salt (sodium and chloride) in it. People without CF have less than 40 milliequivalents/liter (mEq/L) of chloride in their sweat (and a similar concentration of sodium), whereas people with CF have more than 60 mEq/L (and usually more than 80 mEq/L). This means that an analysis of the sweat can tell physicians whether someone has CF or not. Once a test is positive, it will always be positive (meaning that if someone has CF, he or she will always have it). Also, a test is either positive or negative; there are no differences between someone whose sweat chloride concentration is 83 mEq/L and someone whose is 115 mEq/L. The higher number does not mean a worse case of CF.

The Sweat Test

Informal sweat testing has been done for centuries. There was a folk belief in Europe in the Middle Ages that "a child who tastes salty from a kiss on the brow . . . is hexed, and soon must die." Modern day parents of children with CF frequently notice that their babies taste salty when they are kissed and that their older children have salt crystals on their faces and in their hair when they are active in the summertime. However, not everyone's taste buds are sensitive enough to distinguish between CF sweat and non-CF sweat.

Since the 1950's, a more accurate method of sweat testing has been available. The **Gibson–Cooke** method is a sweat test that is highly accurate. When sweat testing is done by any other method, mistakes frequently arise, resulting in "false positives" (children who *don't* have CF but whose tests indicate that they *do* have it) and in "false negatives" (children who *do* have CF but whose tests indicate that they *don't* have it). The correct method, and currently the only acceptable method, is the Gibson–Cooke method of sweat testing by *pilocarpine iontophoresis with quantitative analysis of sodium and/or chloride.*

The Gibson–Cooke method employs the chemical **pilocarpine** to stimulate the sweat glands to produce sweat. Pilocarpine reaches the working part of the sweat gland by first being placed on the skin, and then directed into the sweat gland by a small electrical current; this process is called iontophoresis. The sweat is then collected on a cloth or paper pad, or in a tiny coiled tube. It is then weighed carefully, and the sodium and/or chloride contents are measured very precisely (quantitatively).

To perform the test and collect the sweat takes 30–60 minutes. The laboratory analysis takes another 30 minutes or so. Therefore, it's usually several hours between the time someone comes into the lab and the time the results are ready.

The first step in the test is that the forearm (or occasionally, in a small baby, the lower leg, or even the back) is washed off, to remove anything which might have any salt in it. Then some pilocarpine is placed on the skin. Pilocarpine is colorless and odorless, and looks and feels like water. Two flat metal electrodes are placed on the skin and connected to a small box which sends a slight electrical current (approximately 2–5 milliamps) into the skin, driving the pilocarpine into the vicinity of the sweat gland, where it can "turn on" the sweat gland. The electrical current is usually not felt at all, but some people feel a mild tingling, and a few may even feel a harsher tingling or burning. It should not burn, and if it does, you should tell the technician, so that the current can be turned down.

After about 5 minutes with the electrodes in place, they are removed, the arm (or leg or back) is again wiped off, and a piece of absorbent material (gauze or filter paper) or a tiny coiled tube is placed on the skin. The technician then wraps the arm, covering the gauze with a dressing that is airtight and water-tight, so that no sweat will evaporate or leak out. During the next 30–60 minutes, the dressing is left in place while the "revved up" sweat glands are making sweat. The technician then removes the dressing with tweezers or forceps, taking care not to touch the gauze or filter paper with his or her fingers, puts the paper (now soaked with sweat) into a bottle, and takes it to the lab. In the lab, the technician weighs the bottle to see how much sweat there is, rinses the sweat out of the paper or gauze into a container, and then puts it through the chemical analyzers to find out precisely how much sodium and/or chloride is in the sweat. Some laboratories measure the chloride, some measure the sodium, and some measure both. As long as the sweat is obtained by this method, it doesn't matter which part of the salt is measured.

When the test is performed by this method, *by a laboratory experienced in performing this test,* the result should enable the physician to make a definite and accurate diagnosis.

Problems with Sweat Testing

In an experienced lab, not getting enough sweat is the only major problem that can interfere with obtaining a reliable result. Most lab experts say that they must have 100 mg of sweat in order to be able to do an accurate analysis. Some people, especially very young babies (under 1 month old) may not make enough sweat to analyze. If enough sweat is collected, the results will be valid, even within the first weeks of life, and even in a premature infant.

Adults have higher sweat sodium and chloride levels than children, but even in adults, a sweat chloride concentration greater than 60 mEq/L is abnormal.

There are a very few conditions which give elevated sweat chloride or sodium levels, and these are usually readily distinguished from CF. Similarly, there are very few people with CF whose sweat sodium and chloride concentrations are below 60 mEq/L.

That a hospital or laboratory says they can perform a sweat test is not adequate assurance that they can do it correctly. *Nearly one-half of all patients who come to CF centers having had sweat tests done in outlying hospitals have received incorrect results from these tests.*

Salt Loss

In addition to making the sweat test possible, the sweat abnormality can also affect the health of some people with CF. For each drop of sweat made, considerably more sodium and chloride are lost from the body than would be lost in someone without CF. In most children and adults with CF, the body is able to regulate the amount of salt in the bloodstream amazingly well. When more salt is lost, people want and take in more salt; the kidneys reduce the amount of salt lost through the urine, and so on. Under most circumstances, even including active exercise in hot weather, if adequate salt is available, children and adults with CF will take in the proper amounts. Pretzel sticks and other salty snacks may be available for toddlers, whereas older children and adults can have access to the salt shaker, and no further supplements are needed. Salt tablets are not needed.

Infants with CF may lose too much salt in their sweat, and are not able to let their parents know that they feel like having a pickle or pretzel or other salty food. Each year, especially during summer months, some infants with CF become ill because of having lost too much salt. They become lethargic, their appetite falls off, and they seem sickly. If this happens, they may require hospitalization and intravenous fluids containing replacement sodium and chloride. In order to prevent this problem, it's advisable for infants to be given a tiny bit of salt in their bottles during hot summer months. An amount as small as ⅛ tsp., once or twice a day, is probably adequate. Since too much salt can cause problems, it's best to provide *moderate,* regular supplements.

Some older children and adults who are very active during hot weather will need to be careful about replacing lost fluid and salt. The only immediate danger for a teenager under extreme exertion, such as marathon running or a long, tough football practice in full uniform in hot weather, is fluid loss. Athletes should drink more water than they feel they need, since thirst is not as sensitive a guide as is the taste for salt. Salt replacement does not need to be immediate, and will be accurately guided by taste.

REPRODUCTIVE SYSTEM IN CYSTIC FIBROSIS

Although the reproductive systems of people with CF are basically normal, the thick mucus found in so many other places in the body also affects this system.

The Male Reproductive System in Cystic Fibrosis

In boys and men with CF, the reproductive system is completely normal, with one exception. In 98 percent of boys and men with CF, the **vas deferens** is incompletely formed or totally blocked. The vas deferens is the tube that carries sperm from the testicles to the penis. This is the tube that is cut and tied when a man has a vasectomy. The sperm are normally formed in the testicles, but because of the blockage, they cannot be released. Men with CF have completely normal sex lives, but the 98 percent of these men who have this blockage are sterile. (It is very much as though everything had been normal, and they had gotten a vasectomy.) A small proportion of men with CF (about 2 percent) are not sterile, and some have fathered children.

It is possible to test whether a teenager or adult with CF is one of the 98 percent who are sterile, or one of the 2 percent who are not. The patient simply gives a semen specimen to the lab, where it is analyzed for sperm.

The Female Reproductive System in Cystic Fibrosis

In women with CF, the problems related to the reproductive system are more subtle than in men. The main problem is that the mucus lining the cervix (the opening to the uterus, or womb) is thick, just like mucus elsewhere. As a result it is harder for women with CF to get pregnant than for women without CF. It certainly is possible though, and several hundred women with CF have gotten pregnant, and many of these women have delivered babies.

Women whose lungs are in excellent shape when they get pregnant usually do well with the pregnancy. Women whose lungs are at all involved with CF lung disease may have a very hard time with the pregnancy. There are many women with CF who have been in fairly good health before they became pregnant, but whose health deteriorated during the pregnancy.

Delayed Development

Both boys and girls with CF may go through puberty 1–2 years later than their classmates. This occurs as an indirect result of CF, and is likely to be a direct result of poor nutrition or of chronic lung infection. Delayed development can be a problem in any chronic illness, for energy expended to fight the illness depletes the body's energy reserve for growth. The treatment for this problem is directed at the underlying causes, and in CF that means treating the lungs and improving the nutrition.

4 / Nutrition

Susan R. Orenstein, Margaret F. Gloninger,
and David M. Orenstein

THE IMPORTANCE OF NUTRITION IN CYSTIC FIBROSIS

Malnourished people do not grow well, and often they do not feel well. Malnutrition damages the immune system, which is the body's defense against infection, and, in someone with cystic fibrosis (CF), may contribute to the pulmonary disease and hasten death. Cystic fibrosis patients who are better nourished grow better, have better pulmonary function, and live longer than patients with poor nutrition.

EVALUATION OF NUTRITION

In an adult, generalized malnutrition shows up first as weight loss. In children, who should grow and gain weight actively, a slowing down of the normal weight gain may be the first sign of malnutrition. This is most easily detected by plotting a child's weight on a growth chart (Fig. 4.1). If the child's growth does not keep up with the curves, malnutrition may be the cause.

When malnutrition affects growth, it usually affects weight first of all. When weight has been severely affected, height may begin to show signs of falling behind the growth curves. Finally, if severe malnutrition affects a very young child at a time when the brain is actively growing, the head circumference growth may decrease. These three measurements should be plotted regularly for children, in order to identify signs of malnutrition or other health problems when they begin, before you might notice them in the children's appearance.

Another method of assessing general nutritional state is called *anthropometrics* ("measuring people"). Measurements are taken such as skin-fold thickness, which determines how much fat is stored in the body (a certain amount of such fat storage is normal and desirable), and mid-arm muscle circumference, which is a measure of protein stored in the body in muscles.

Many aspects of a person's nutritional state can also be measured by

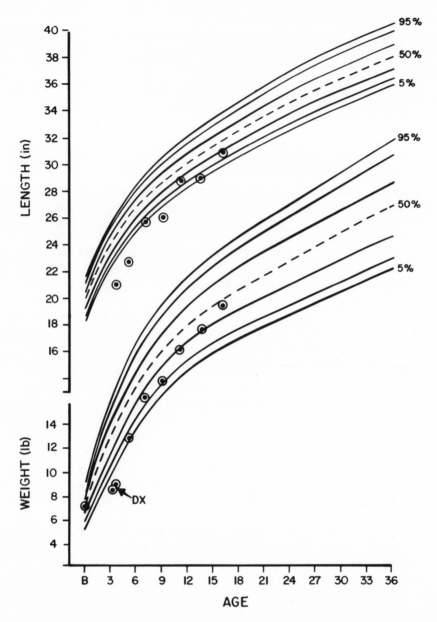

FIG. 4.1. Growth chart. The *solid lines* represent the length and weight growth curves for normal children at various ages (in months). The "5%" line refers to the length and weight of healthy children in the lowest 5 percent for their age: that is, 5 percent of healthy children will have a weight that falls on or below the 5% line, whereas 95 percent will be heavier. The "50%" *dotted lines* represent the 50th percentile, or the average length and weight for healthy children. The *circles* represent the specific measurements for one youngster with CF. This child's weight was near average at birth (B), and fell below the 5th percentile by the time of diagnosis (DX). Treatment began after diagnosis, and the child's weight reached just below the average by age at 18 months.

blood tests such as albumin, total protein, triglycerides, cholesterol, carotene, glucose, and hemoglobulin.

CAUSES OF MALNUTRITION IN CYSTIC FIBROSIS

At one time it was assumed that the malnutrition that affects so many children and adults with CF was entirely due to the poor digestion of food, which, in turn, was due to the lack of pancreatic enzymes and bile salts, as was discussed in Chapter 2. Though enzyme deficiency is a major cause of malnutrition in CF (and has been greatly relieved by the availability of enzyme replacement), there are additional contributing factors to malnutrition: (1) enzyme supplements do not work perfectly, (2) people with CF may not take in enough calories, even for someone with normal needs, and (3) there are increased caloric needs in CF.

Enzyme Deficiency

Although the enzymes help a great deal, they are not usually completely effective. Given as capsules with the meal, they may not arrive in the duodenum at the precise time to meet up with the food. The inaccuracy of enzyme supplements is due to the difficulty of mimicking perfectly the body's finely tuned system for trickling the pancreatic juice in just as the food arrives. Enzymes also may be inactivated in the stomach by stomach acid; this probably happens to 80–90 percent of the nonenteric-coated enzymes taken. We do not usually supplement bile salts, so this may prevent the enzymes we give from acting optimally. Finally, in CF the pancreatic bicarbonate is not secreted very well, and therefore stomach acid is not completely neutralized. This may prevent the enteric coating of enzymes from dissolving.

Inadequate Caloric Intake

In addition to the imperfect supplementation of pancreatic enzymes, the poor caloric intake of many people with CF contributes to their malnutrition. It is commonly believed that people with CF have a large appetite, and some do. But many children, teenagers, and adults with CF actually eat less food than their friends. Malnutrition itself may decrease a person's appetite (this is called the "anorexia of malnutrition"). Feeling sick and coughing a lot also decrease a person's appetite. In addition, previous nutritional recommendations for CF patients have been confusing: for a period of time it was believed that a low fat diet should be taken by CF patients because the bowel movements appeared better if there was less fat in them. Though less fat in the diet does mean less fat in the stools, unfortunately, it also means fewer calories in the body as a whole. Low fat diets attempt to make up for the lost fat calories by increasing carbohydrate calories. However, an ounce of fat has more than twice the energy (calories) present in an ounce of carbohydrate, so if you are on a low fat diet you have to eat a lot more to get the same number of calories for growth. On a low fat diet many people with CF were therefore unable to take in enough calories. With recent improvements in enzyme therapy, *a low fat diet is no longer recommended* except under very special circumstances.

Increased Caloric Needs

The third reason for malnutrition in CF is an *increased use* of calories. Coughing and breathing hard require extra calories. If you are using extra calories in this way all day long, the need for extra calories accumulates. Even fighting lung infections requires extra calories.

SPECIAL DEFICIENCIES IN CYSTIC FIBROSIS

Hypoalbuminemia (Low Blood Albumin Levels)

Albumin is the main body protein in blood. One of its primary roles in the blood is to keep water in the arteries and veins. If there is not enough albumin in the blood, water leaks out into the skin and other organs, and produces skin puffiness called *edema*. Hypoalbuminemia and edema may occur in infants with CF before they are diagnosed, and may be the clue that leads to diagnosis of CF. It is more likely to show up, and to show up earlier in infants fed soy milk, because soy formulas may not provide the protein reserve that the cow milk formulas do. Hypoalbuminemia is treated by giving pancreatic enzymes and plenty of protein in the diet. Some infants with very low blood albumin also benefit from several intravenous injections of albumin, which provides them with albumin before they are able to begin making it themselves out of the protein in their diet.

Essential Fatty Acid Deficiency

Fatty acids are the parts of the fat (triglyceride) molecule. Essential fatty acids are fatty acids that the body needs and which it cannot make from other nutrients. Two essential fatty acids, linoleic acid and linolenic acid, are found in all dietary fats and are also abundant in plant oils such as safflower, corn, and sunflower oils. These are needed for a number of complex and necessary functions, including the manufacture of cell membranes. They also appear to be needed for optimal lung function. The difficulties in fat digestion and absorption in CF can show up early as deficiencies of these essential fatty acids, since the body's needs for them cannot be met by making them out of other nutrients. In addition, the essential fatty acids that do get absorbed may get used for other caloric needs: for example, they get "burned up" to supply energy for breathing. This deficiency can be treated by increasing the caloric intake, and by taking special supplements such as safflower oil.

Fat-Soluble Vitamins (Vitamins A, D, E, and K)

These four vitamins are often at low levels in patients with CF. This may be in part because these vitamins are found with dietary fat that is not absorbed well. It is difficult to determine the best dose of supplemental vitamins for a particular patient, so CF patients are often put on a "standard" dose, which is higher than that recommended for people without CF. A physical examination (and sometimes blood tests) can then tell if more vitamins are required. It is very important for people not to take "megadoses" of these vitamins from a health food store, without a physician's guidance, since these vitamins can be dangerous if taken in too large quantities.

Vitamin A

Vitamin A is needed for vision and growth. Retinol and carotene are two types of vitamin A. Vitamin A is found in animal products, especially liver and fortified milk. Carotene is found in dark green and deep yellow vegetables and in fruit, and is converted to active vitamin A in the body. Vitamin A is normally absorbed from the intestine and then stored in the liver to be used when it is needed. Two proteins made by the liver—prealbumin and retinol-binding protein—are needed to extract the vitamin A from the liver. In people with CF, blood levels of vitamin A are below normal even when supplemental enzymes and vitamin A are given, but they are usually not so low that they produce symptoms. The abnormal fat digestion is part of the problem with vitamin A in CF, but even when vitamin A is absorbed and stored in the liver, it will not be available to the body if there are low levels of prealbumin and retinol-binding protein. The reason for the low levels of these two proteins in CF is unknown.

Vitamin D

Vitamin D is needed to get the minerals calcium and phosphorus from the diet into blood, where they are needed for growth of bones and for normal functioning of many other organs. Low levels of vitamin D cause a bone disease called *rickets,* in which the bones are abnormally soft. Vitamin D is found in fortified milk and dairy products. It is also made in the skin by the action of sunlight. Vitamin D from the diet or skin must then be activated by the liver and kidneys, which means that people with liver disease or kidney disease are more susceptible to vitamin D deficiency. Rickets or other evidence of vitamin D deficiency is rare in CF, particularly when patients are given supplemental pancreatic enzymes and vitamin D. If it does occur, it can be detected by blood tests and treated with special supplemental vitamin and mineral preparations; plenty of sunshine is also helpful.

Vitamin E

Vitamin E is important for the functioning of a number of important body parts, especially nerves. It is found in vegetable oil, whole grains, and eggs. Symptoms of vitamin E deficiency may include unsteadiness while walking. Vitamin E deficiency also causes an abnormal knee jerk reflex, which the doctor checks by hitting the knee with the rubber hammer. Vitamin E deficiency can be detected by blood tests. If these tests indicate a deficiency, a higher dose of vitamin E can be given. Water-soluble forms of the vitamins are much easier to absorb than most health food store preparations of vitamin E.

Vitamin K

Vitamin K is needed by the liver for making some of the clotting factors that stop bleeding. Green leafy vegetables are good food sources of vitamin K and it is also found in fruits, dairy products, and meats. The average diet provides enough vitamin K so that no supplement is needed. It is also made by bacteria that normally live in the intestines. But in the CF patient, vitamin K may not be well absorbed. If blood levels of vitamin K are too low, very serious bleeding can result. There are several blood tests for clotting; the most common are the "PT" test (prothrombin time) and the "PTT" test (partial thromboplastin time). The PT becomes abnormal if levels of vitamin K are too low. This can be corrected by increasing the amount of vitamin taken, either in the form of pills or by injection. Since the liver is needed to make the clotting factors, even vitamin K given by injection may not provide enough if the liver is failing to work (as in severe cirrhosis, discussed in Chapter 2). In this case, the already-made clotting factors may be given by giving a kind of transfusion of "fresh frozen plasma."

Hypomagnesemia

Magnesium, like calcium, phosphorus, sodium, and chloride, is one of the minerals the body needs. Good food sources of magnesium include dark green leafy vegetables and dairy products. Normally, magnesium is absorbed from the diet, and the kidneys put any extra magnesium out in the urine. When there is too little magnesium in the blood (hypomagnesemia) the signs include weakness, shakiness, and muscle cramps. In CF, there are a number of causes for hypomagnesemia. Diarrhea may prevent the magnesium from being absorbed from the intestine. Some of the antibiotics given for lung infections (especially the ones ending in "-micin" or "-mycin"), and diuretics given for heart or liver problems may cause too much magnesium to be lost in the urine. Hypomagnesemia can be checked for during the physical examination: the knee-jerk reflexes are too brisk (the opposite of what happens with vitamin E deficiency) and tests of the hand and face muscles show muscle spasms. Blood measurement of magnesium helps make the diagnosis of hypomagnesemia. Treatment is by oral or intravenous magnesium supplements.

Hypoelectrolytemia

The main chemicals in the bloodstream that carry an electrical charge, such as sodium, chloride, and potassium, are called *electrolytes*. People with CF lose a lot of salt in their sweat, and since salt consists of sodium and chloride, they may lose enough sodium and chloride to lower the blood levels of these electrolytes. This is especially likely to happen during exertion in hot weather, or in infants, who can't choose their own diet.

Once CF is diagnosed, the problem can usually be prevented, and most CF physicians advise parents to put a small amount of salt (⅛ teaspoon) in each bottle for their babies with CF during the hot months. This small amount will prevent the problem from developing, and will also avoid the serious problems which could be seen by giving too much salt. Older children need no special treatment, other than free access to salty foods or the salt shaker. They will know how much salt to take.

This problem is discussed in Chapter 3.

NUTRITIONAL TREATMENT

Basic Nutritional Treatment

Basic nutritional treatment in CF consists of a well-rounded diet with plenty of protein, carbohydrate, and fat taken with enough pancreatic enzymes to provide maximum absorption. Tables 4.1 and 4.2 contain guidelines and suggestions for maintaining good nutritional intake. The caloric intake required to maintain good growth is usually between one-and-a-third and one-and-a-half times that required for a person of the same age and sex without CF. Table salt and salty foods may be used liberally. Supplemental fat-soluble vitamins are given each day, and periodic checking is done to

TABLE 4.1. *Dietary guidelines*

1. **Protein intake** should be increased to provide the building blocks used by the body to build body tissue. Protein is supplied in the diet by such foods as meat, fish, poultry, dairy products, eggs, legumes, and peanut butter.

2. **Additional fats** should be included in the diet, primarily in the form of vegetable oils. Fats have a high concentration of calories.

3. **Low bulk carbohydrates,** such as starches and sugars, also have a high concentration of calories and should be increased. Carbohydrates are easily digested.

4. **Fruits and vegetables** should be included in the diet for variety as well as to supply important nutrients. Excessive amounts of high bulk foods should be avoided, as these foods tend to make a person feel full without supplying many calories.

5. **High calorie, nutritious snacks** are a *must.*

6. **Special formula products** (see Table 4.3) are available in pharmacies and some supermarkets and are helpful as supplements to increase calories. Some of these formulas contain enough nutrients for a totally balanced meal. However, they should not be taken in place of a regular meal except during an acute illness if no other food is tolerated.

TABLE 4.2. *Suggestions for parents for improving their child's nutrition*[a]

Do's
1. Plan a definite eating schedule with three well-balanced meals and at least two snacks daily.
2. In order that snacks not lessen the appetite for the next meal, offer snacks *after,* not before, meals.
3. Give a large, high calorie snack at bedtime. [If the child has problems with reflux (see Chapter 2) the last snack should be a bit before bedtime.]
4. Make foods attractive to encourage the child to eat.
5. Try to increase the size of servings.
6. Try to get the child to drink at least one quart of whole milk daily, or, better yet, a high nutrient milkbase drink such as a milkshake.
7. Fortify quick breads, mashed potatoes, milk desserts, juices, and whole milk with extra nonfat, dry-milk solids and/or polycose.
8. Serve bread with a generous amount of a spread such as cream cheese, peanut butter, margarine, or jelly.
9. Offer juices or nectars instead of water (water has no calories).
10. Serve bacon or sausage with breakfast.
11. Serve creamed or thickened soup instead of a thin soup.
12. Serve gravy on meat and potatoes.
13. Serve mayonnaise, oil and dressings, and creamed sauces whenever possible with sandwiches, salads, and vegetables.
14. Add sauce or a whipped topping to desserts such as puddings, custards, gelatin, cakes, and ice cream.
15. Offer nuts between meals or add to fruits, salads, and desserts.
16. Praise your child when he or she is eating well.

Don't's
1. Don't nag (it doesn't help).
2. Don't force feed your child (he or she will rebel).
3. Don't get upset if your child doesn't eat. Remove the food quietly and offer it, or a nutritious snack, an hour or so later.
4. Don't fight with your child over eating (the child often wins and no one benefits).

[a]Teenagers and adults can create their own guidelines based on these suggestions.

make sure that these and other aspects of nutrition are adequate. These simple measures usually have a dramatic effect. Babies who were tiny, and could not put on any weight, often will catch up to their growth curve and begin to look much healthier very soon after starting their enzymes (see Fig. 3.1). Occasionally, one of several types of antacid medications (liquid antacids, cimetidine, ranitidine) may be given to help the enzymes work better.

But what if a person eats as much as she or he can, and still is not growing well? Since it is critical to maintain nutrition, the following additions to a well-rounded diet should be considered.

High Calorie Nutritional Supplements

Commercial and homemade (e.g., milkshakes) high calorie nutritional supplements can be prescribed if routine nutritional measures are not sufficient. Sometimes a person who cannot eat enough calories in his or her regular diet can take enough extra calories with these supplements to start gaining properly again. Suggestions for high calorie supplements are presented in Table 4.3 (see page 80).

Tube Feeding

Nutritional supplements can be fed by tube if taking them orally is insufficient. This method involves giving nutritional supplements through a tube that reaches into the gastrointestinal tract. In this way, nutrition can continue during the night while a person sleeps. This has been done for CF patients in a number of different ways. Some patients have used a **nasogastric** tube (or NG tube) that passes in through the nose, down the throat, and into the stomach. Many young children who found this idea repellent at first have quickly gotten used to the tube, and older children have learned to insert the tube themselves each night before bed. The improvement in growth and appearance and feeling of well-being has made this extra effort worth it to them.

A second method of tube feeding is through a **gastrostomy**. In this method a tube is placed through the skin of the upper abdomen and into the stomach during a minor operation. This tube has the advantage of not having to be replaced each night, and it does not involve the discomfort of a tube that goes through the nose. It also does not interfere with breathing or coughing. It is worn under the clothes when not being used, and can be hooked up to the supplemental feeding at night. When it is no longer needed it can simply be removed without an operation.

Jejunostomy feeding is similar to gastrostomy feeding, except the tube goes into the intestine. It is less commonly used, but has the advantage of protecting against gastroesophageal reflux of the tube feeding (see Chapter

TABLE 4.3. *Nutritional supplements*[a]

	Serving size	Calories per serving
Special Formula Products[b]		
Ensure Liquid	8 oz.	250
Ensure Plus Liquid	8 oz.	355
Sustacal Liquid	8 oz.	250
Sustacal Pudding	5 oz.	240
Citrotein	8 oz.	170
Nutrament	12 oz.	360
Polycose Liquid[c]	As desired	30 cal./Tbsp.
Polycose Powder[c]	As desired	30 cal./Tbsp.
High Calorie Foods[d]		
Carnation Instant Breakfast (made with whole milk)	8 oz. (1 cup)	300
Half-and-half	½ cup	160
Ice cream	½ cup	140
Peanut butter	2 Tbsp	180
Hershey New Trail	1 bar	200
Carnation Breakfast Bar	1 bar	200
Macadamia nuts	1 oz.	218
Planter's Nut Mix	1 oz.	180
Whipped cream	¼ cup	103
Mayonnaise	2 Tbsp.	196
Super shake (1 serving)[e]	12 oz.	480

[a]Special formulas as well as regular foods that are naturally high in calories can be used to increase calories. *Remember that fats such as margarine, butter, and oils are high in calories.* Some other foods that are high in fat are ice cream, half-and-half, gravies, salad dressings, meats, nuts, pastries, and peanut butter.

[b]All of these formulas, except Polycose, require enzymes.

[c]Polycose is a sugar supplement. It can be mixed into various foods to increase their calories without changing their taste. It can combine with milk, tea, mashed potatoes, casseroles, or soups.

[d]You can make many different high calorie foods with "double milk." This means that if a dried food package like soup or potatoes calls for adding water, you can add milk instead.

[e]Recipe: 8 oz. whole milk
      4 Tbsp. powdered skim milk
      1 packet Instant Breakfast
      4 oz. vanilla ice cream

2). Predigested formulas are often used for the gastrostomy and jejunostomy feedings. These formulas do not need enzymes for digestion or absorption.

Intravenous Nutrition

Intravenous nutrition is rarely required, because nutritional supplements or tube feeding are usually sufficient to improve nutrition. Intravenous nutrition (also called parenteral nutrition or hyperalimentation) can be given through a long-term IV into a large vein, usually in the upper chest. As with the supplemental nutrition by mouth and by tube, intravenous nutrition can be given at home, so that a person's life can be continued normally.

5// Hospitalization and Other Special Treatments

David M. Orenstein

HOSPITALIZATION

The most common reason for a hospital admission for someone with cystic fibrosis (CF) is treatment of a pulmonary exacerbation (see Chapter 1). This chapter reviews what happens during such a hospitalization. (If someone is admitted to the hospital for another reason, different tests and treatments will be required.)

Admission Procedures

Checking In

There are several procedures that occur routinely in most hospitals when someone is admitted for intensive treatment. One begins at the admissions office where you'll be asked questions and given forms to fill out about insurance. Then you'll go to one of the hospital's inpatient floors where a nurse will ask you questions about your medical history (allergies, usual medications, etc.), weigh and measure you, and check your pulse and temperature. The next step is usually to meet a doctor who will ask more extensive questions about your medical history and then perform a physical examination. In a small community hospital, the doctor may be your own physician; in a large university hospital, the doctor is likely to be an intern or resident (see below for an explanation of the "cast of characters"). After the questions and exam, the physician will write orders for treatment and the necessary medical procedures will begin.

Needles

Most hospitalizations require some painful procedures involving needles. IV's are used to get medications into the bloodstream, and blood tests are taken to make sure the treatment isn't causing problems.

IV for medications

One of the main reasons for being admitted to the hospital is to take the powerful antibiotics (especially those which kill *Pseudomonas*) that are only effective when given directly into the bloodstream. In order to do this, a needle is stuck through the skin into the vein. There are several types of needles that can be used, including metal needles ("butterfly") or plastic catheters ("intracaths," "medicuts," etc.). Whatever type is used, it will hurt a little as it pierces the skin, but once it is in place and is taped down to keep it stable, it is rarely painful. Babies, children, and older patients alike can usually carry on their daily activities with an IV in place.

The veins that are most often used are those on the back of the hands and on the forearms, but if these veins are difficult to find in an infant (as is often the case with a chubby baby), foot veins or veins in the scalp may be used. Foot veins should not be used in anyone who can walk unless there is no other choice. Scalp vein IV's look as though they'd be very uncomfortable, and most parents are bothered by the idea of them at first, but they are no more painful than an arm vein IV and have the advantage of not requiring the immobilization of an arm. If a hand or arm vein is used, an arm-board (which looks like a splint) helps to keep the hand or forearm stable, which in turn helps keep the needle within the vein. A plastic or cardboard cup may be taped over the needle to protect it and prevent it from being bumped.

When the IV is about to be started, it's a good idea to tell the person starting it if you have preferences about which hand or arm to use: If someone is right-handed, it's better to leave the right hand alone, so it can be used to write, play ping-pong, etc. If a baby has favorite fingers or thumb to suck, he or she will be much happier if those fingers or thumb is not taped out of mouth's reach.

Once the needle is in place, the medicines can be given through it. The medications are mixed with saline (salt water) or dextrose (sugar) water and then either allowed to drip through tubing into the IV under the force of gravity, or are pushed through the tubing by electric pumps that regulate precisely how much goes in and how fast. It usually takes about 30–60 minutes for antibiotics to run into the vein. When the medications have finished going into the vein, the needle may then be connected to tubing through which simple saline or dextrose mixtures are passed until it is time for the next antibiotic. A much more convenient procedure is to flush the IV needle with a small amount of saline and heparin (a drug that prevents blood clots from blocking the needle) and then to leave a cap on the end of the needle. Once the needle is flushed with heparin and capped, it can safely be left alone for many hours and will be ready for use when it's time to give the next dose of antibiotics. This means that the person does not have to be tied continually to the IV apparatus of tubing and bottles, and will be free to move about.

Blood tests

When someone is admitted to the hospital, several kinds of blood tests are usually done. Almost always, these admission tests can be done with one needle stick, even if several tubes of blood are needed (the total amount of blood needed will seldom be more than one tablespoon). Different tests may be done, including blood counts and measurement of blood electrolytes (chemicals such as sodium, chloride, and potassium). It is also common to check the blood levels of chemicals that reflect kidney function, since many antibiotics can affect kidney function.

Some of the tests are done only at admission, but others are repeated periodically through the hospitalization. For example, kidney function tests might be repeated once or twice a week to make sure that the drugs have not caused a problem. Blood may be taken several times to measure antibiotic levels. This is done especially to check on the aminoglycoside antibiotics (see *Appendix B: Medications*). The effectiveness of these medicines probably relates to the peak level of the drug (the highest level that is reached), and their toxicity most likely relates to the "trough" (lowest level). Since the peak usually occurs within 30–60 minutes after the medication enters the vein, and the trough is hours later (just before the next dose), careful monitoring of drug levels will necessitate a double test, one just after the drug has gone in, and one just before the next dose. If the levels are too low or too high, the physicians will know that they must adjust the dose. In this way, it is possible to get the maximum benefit from the medications and the minimum toxicity. At the same time it's a bother, since blood levels must be checked again. Once the right dose is found, however, it is not necessary to recheck the levels frequently.

Other tests

Chest X-rays and pulmonary function tests, perhaps including a blood gas test, may also be done shortly after admission and at intervals during the hospitalization, in order to monitor the progress you are making (see Chapter 1 for a discussion of these tests). Electrocardiogram (ECG) and echocardiograms are often performed in order to determine the heart's condition and to estimate how much stress it is under. Other tests might also be done depending on the circumstances. A hearing test might be performed if drugs are being used that might affect hearing. As always, if you do not understand what a test is, or why it's being done, ask.

Treatment

Medicines

The main part of the hospital treatment of worsened lung infection is IV antibiotics. Two different antibiotics are commonly used. Each of the antibiotics must be given on its own schedule. Schedules range from every 4 hours to every 12 hours, with the most common intervals being every 6 or 8 hours. If blood levels are checked, they may indicate that the schedule needs to be changed, for example, from every 8 hours to every 6 hours. Other aspects of the treatment will vary at different CF centers, but will often include chest physical therapy two to four times a day (or even more), aerosol treatments, vitamins, pancreatic enzymes, and plenty of calories. Anti-inflammatory medications (e.g., prednisone) may be included in the treatment. Exercise may or may not be prescribed, but in most cases, patients should be up and out of bed most of the day. In some hospitals, you may be able to attend school (your own school or an in-hospital school room) or work on an altered schedule built around the medication schedules.

Length of Stay

The ideal length of time to get IV antibiotics to fight bronchial infection is the time it takes to get you back to your baseline pulmonary function, that is, the amount of time needed to get you back to your usual state of health. Most often, this is approximately 2 weeks, but it can easily take 3 weeks. It is rarely more than 3 weeks or less than 2. Most CF experts feel that it is a mistake to let the calendar determine the length of treatment without regard to the patient's progress; rather, it is the patient's response to treatment that should dictate the length of hospitalization. Pulmonary function tests (PFT's) and a physical examination can often help in determining the length of stay, but often it is the patients themselves and their families who contribute most to this decision. They are the people who know best, for example, just how much the patient is coughing. The observations of the patient and family are very important in this regard. While several weeks in the hospital can seem like a very long time, and it may be tempting to try to arrange discharge as early as possible, it is wise to remember that the time invested in achieving good health is time well spent. It is quite possible that a few extra days at the end of a hospitalization may mean several weeks or months of good health.

Complications

As with any treatment, hospitalization can have some bad effects along with the good. These may be emotional, psychological, or educational, as might be expected if a child has to miss several weeks of school and contact with friends. Being removed from familiar surroundings, experiencing painful procedures, and having very little control over one's environment can be upsetting, especially to a toddler who may understand only the pain and not the explanation that it is necessary to help him or her get well again. It takes time after discharge for one's life to return to normal, but with patience and understanding, it always does.

Some specific in-hospital complications should be anticipated. IV's last only for a limited period, for they eventually go bad ("infiltrate") and need to be replaced: antibiotics are powerful chemicals, and may irritate the vein, eventually weakening its wall so that it starts to leak and swell and becomes tender. When this happens, it is time for a new IV. Although IV's may occasionally last a couple of weeks, a few days is closer to the average. Rarely, there may be other complications such as evidence of kidney damage from the antibiotics. It is to spot these complications that the blood tests are periodically performed. Once the problem is spotted, stopping or reducing the antibiotics nearly always eliminates kidney problems.

Daily Life in the Hospital

Most often when CF patients are admitted to the hospital for treatment of a pulmonary exacerbation, they are not terribly sick or disabled. The reason for these hospitalizations is to *keep someone relatively well,* and not to cure someone who is dreadfully ill. Some people, including young doctors or nurses may not understand that and may even say, "you don't look sick enough to be in the hospital." They miss the point that your health is suffering and that the reason for the hospitalization is to get you back to your normal state of good health. While you probably won't be so sick that you need to be in bed all day, it is important to remember that you are in the hospital to improve your present and future health.

What to Wear

You will probably be up and around most of the day, so you should wear regular clothes. It is not necessary for pajamas or hospital gowns to make an appearance between breakfast and bedtime.

Activity

You should try not to let being in the hospital decrease your activity. Most hospitals, especially children's hospitals, will have playrooms and teen lounges, and you should take advantage of these facilities. You may be able to use a physical therapy gym, or even to leave the hospital (on a pass) to get even more activity. This may be a chance to visit museums or other favorite places. Once again, *you should not lie in bed all day.*

School Work

Two or three weeks is a lot of time to miss from the school year, so it is very important to try to keep up with your school work. Your doctor can help you arrange for work to be sent or brought to you in the hospital. Some hospitals have a schoolteacher on their staff to help students keep up with work. Some school systems have arrangements for home (or hospital) tutors for anyone who will be out of school a certain amount of time. It is very important that you do whatever is necessary to keep up with school work while you're in the hospital.

The "Cast of Characters"

You will meet many different people in the hospital in addition to other patients, and it can be confusing as you try to figure out who everybody is. Remember, with any problems or major questions, your doctor is in charge.

Nurses and Aides

Hospitals could not run without nurses and aides. They will check you in, check your "vital signs" (pulse, respiratory rate, temperature, etc.), give you your medications, and in general help to make your stay successful and pleasant. They may be able to answer many of the questions that arise regarding treatments, schedules, etc. The nursing staff probably does more than everyone else combined to make your stay a positive (or, in very rare cases, a negative) experience.

Physicians

You are likely to see a number of different physicians in addition to your own doctor. Especially if you are in a children's hospital and/or a teaching hospital, you will also be meeting a number of people at the various levels of medical training. It is helpful to know the different stages of medical training.

Medical students have gone to college for four years and are now enrolled in a 4-year medical school. The first 2 years consist of classroom learning. In the third and fourth years, students spend time in the hospital learning the various specialties such as pediatrics, general internal medicine, and surgery. After completing 4 years of medical school, students graduate and get their doctoral degree (M.D.). They are now doctors.

The first step after becoming a doctor is internship. An **intern** is a doctor who is beginning to train in one specialty—pediatrics, internal medicine, family medicine, surgery, psychiatry, or obstetrics/gynecology. After the internship year, the specialty training continues with 2–4 years of "residency." (Most programs no longer call first-year trainees "interns," but rather, "first-year **residents**.") After a resident has finished the three-year residency, he or she is qualified to set up practice as a specialist (family doctor, pediatrician, etc.).

Some physicians choose to get even more specialized training, and take 2 or 3-year subspecialty fellowships. Subspecialties include pulmonology (respiratory problems), cardiology (heart), and neurosurgery (brain and nervous system surgery). Some of the "trainees" you meet might be young students, whereas others may have had 4 years of college, 4 years of medical school, 3 years of pediatric or medicine residencies, and several years of fellowship.

Interacting with many different people at various levels of training and understanding can be difficult for patients and families, especially when several people ask you the same questions. It may also be frustrating to realize that you know more about CF than some of the nurses and physicians who will be taking care of you or your child. Remember, though, that your own physician is knowledgeable about CF and is in charge of your (or your child's) treatment.

In addition, you can view this as an opportunity to help in the education of the people who will be the nurses and physicians in the community. Many families with a child with CF have had the very frustrating experience of going from doctor to doctor trying to find out what was wrong until they found one who knew about CF. One of the best things that anyone can do to help future children with CF is to make a contribution to the education of physicians who will be seeing those children, so that eventually all family doctors, pediatricians, and even adult medical specialists will be knowledgeable about CF, will be able to recognize it, and will have an idea of how to begin treatment.

Consultants

Occasionally, your physician may ask a colleague to give an opinion about a problem or a possible treatment. The other physician will probably look through your chart, ask some questions, and do a physical exam. This colleague is likely to be a specialist or subspecialist, possibly, a gastroenterologist (stomach, liver, and digestive system specialist), surgeon, or cardiologist. These colleagues who are called in to give an opinion about one part of the treatment plan are called *consultants*. It is the job of the consultant to

give an opinion and perhaps make suggestions. It is not the consultant's job
to carry out treatments or order tests without your physician's approval.

Other Health Professionals

In addition to nurses and physicians, you are likely to have contact with
other professionals, including physical therapists and respiratory therapists,
who may be involved with your aerosols and postural drainage treatments.
Some hospitals will have child-life workers to help make the hospitalization
a more positive experience. These people are trained in child development
principles, and are frequently clever at finding just the right kind of entertainment for a child in the strange environment of the hospital. More importantly, they are sensitive to the signals children give through their play and
talk about things that are upsetting or threatening to them. Child-life workers
and child development specialists often can give parents, nurses, and physicians important insights into what is going on in the minds of hospitalized
children.

Nutritionists or dieticians may help with menu selection. Social workers
will be available to help with a variety of problems, from very tough family
adjustment problems (these are discussed in Chapter 9) to the day-to-day
worries of insurance and transportation expenses. Other people you may
come in contact with include people from a TV service, hospital maintenance people, and janitors.

BRINGING THE HOSPITAL HOME

There are many ways that complex and even invasive kinds of treatment
can be carried out at home, thus avoiding prolonged hospitalization. These
include home IV's, various kinds of tube feedings, and different ways of
giving oxygen.

Home IV's

Intravenous treatments are useful especially for getting antibiotics into the
bloodstream to treat worsened bronchial infection (pulmonary exacerbations). In most cases, this treatment is done in the hospital, but in some
cases, once it is clear that progress is being made, it can be completed at
home. Several things must be taken care of before someone can be sent
home with an IV: there must be someone at home to take care of the IV—
to connect the tubing to the needle for infusing the antibiotics, to flush the
tubing and needle after the antibiotics have run in, and to keep the needle
from clogging. The medications must be mixed and stored properly, and they

must be run in at the right speed. Someone must be available who knows what to do if the IV comes out or goes bad. Arrangements also have to be made for regular checkups, including blood tests (antibiotic levels, etc., as would be necessary in the hospital) and physician exams.

Who Takes Care of the IV?

In many metropolitan areas, home medical care companies have taken on many of the tasks of visiting homes, helping to restart IV's when necessary, working with families to run the IV medications, supplying electric pumps to regulate the speed at which the medication is run in, drawing blood for tests, working with pharmacies to supply the medications, and so on. If such a service is not available, public health organizations, such as Visiting Nurses, may help with these details. In other cases, families and physicians have been able to piece together a team of people to do the various things. Some emergency room nurses have volunteered to restart IV's when necessary, and helpful pharmacists may take care of preparing the antibiotics.

Checking Up

Once someone is freed from the constraints of the hospital, it is easy to forget that if he or she were in the hospital, there would be physicians to monitor the progress of the treatment and to check for evidence of drug toxicity at least once a day. It is important to maintain close contact with your physician after hospitalization, particularly if you're still taking the powerful drugs which traditionally have been given only under supervision in a hospital. Checkups once a week, or more or less frequently, may be necessary.

Home IV's for Prolonged Use: The Central Line

In a few patients, IV antibiotics (or rarely, other IV treatment) may be needed very frequently or for a prolonged time. In these cases, it is not convenient or comfortable to keep using regular hand or arm vein IV's which only last a few days before they have to be changed. In these cases, a "long line," or a "central line," can be lifesaving, or at least much more convenient. These lines are a special kind of IV that has its end in a very large vein, or in the heart. When this IV is used, the medication runs into an area of very large blood flow, so that even powerful chemicals will be diluted quickly and will not irritate the veins the way they do with a hand vein. Long lines are usually tunneled under the skin (and in some cases, placed *entirely* under the skin) so that they will not accidentally become dislodged.

The three main types of central lines are Broviac catheters, Hickman catheters, and Mediports (or Infusaports). The Hickman and Broviac catheters are similar, and are lines that are inserted through a small incision, usually in the skin of the neck or by the collarbone, with one end being placed in one of the large veins in the neck, and threaded down into the superior vena cava (the largest vein bringing blood back to the heart from the upper part of the body) or into the heart itself, while the other end may be tunneled under the skin of the chest. In this way, the only part of the catheter that is in contact with the external environment (air, clothes, bath water, etc.) is the tip, which comes out from under the skin on the front or side of the chest. Once the original incisions have healed completely, it's safe to bathe, play sports, and pursue normal activities with the line in place. You should avoid getting hit directly in the chest, and some surgeons prefer that you not swim with one of these long lines in place, but everyone agrees that most normal activities are perfectly safe. The Mediports and Infusaports go entirely under the skin, so any activity (other than those in which the area would be hit hard) is safe with these devices.

Placement of Long Line IV's

Most of the long lines are placed by surgeons; but some particularly skillful pediatricians or internists might also do the line placement. Depending on the age and nervousness of the patient, either a sedative or general anesthesia is given, and if the patient is awake, the areas of incisions will be numbed with injections of local anesthetics (e.g., Novocain). Most often, these procedures are performed while the patient is in the hospital, but recovery from the procedure is very rapid.

Equipment

Some special equipment is needed for the proper care and use of the central lines, especially when they are used out of the hospital. Supplies for keeping them sterile are essential. Special pumps are helpful to push medications in at the proper rate, since problems could develop with medications running in too fast or too slowly. Special needles and tubing are needed to attach the central lines to the bottle or plastic bag holding the medication. For Hickman and Broviac catheters, the needles pierce the rubber cap at the end of the line, but for the Infusaports and Mediports, special needles are required to pierce the skin and stay firmly in the reservoir under the skin. Solutions must be on hand to flush the lines after use (these typically contain saline and heparin to keep blood clots from forming in the line while it's not being used).

Care of Central Lines

Exquisite care must be taken so that these lines do not become infected. Infection in these lines nearly always means that they must be removed. If they need to be replaced, another procedure is required and perhaps another session under general anesthesia, entailing additional risks. More importantly, these lines are in the heart or close to it, and infection in the lines means serious bloodstream infection in the patient. People can get extremely ill from bloodstream infection. Fortunately, with proper care, these lines seldom become infected, even out of the hospital, perhaps because the people who take care of the lines at home are usually the patients themselves or a close family member. Whenever the small dressing (often little more than a Band-Aid) is changed, and medications begun, the technique used must be sterile (allowing no germs to enter). Sterile gloves are worn, the area is cleaned according to strict guidelines, using strong antiseptic solutions, and all tubing ends which would touch the end of the central line are kept scrupulously clean.

Care must also be taken to see that the lines are not pulled out or bumped hard. This protection is easy to provide: the tubes are quite thin and only a short portion sticks out of the skin, so the tubing can be coiled and covered with a small amount of gauze and taped in place. Care of the central lines that are totally under the skin (Mediports, Infusaports) is easier between courses of medication than care of the lines with ends sticking out from under the skin. In fact, other than avoiding direct hits to the site of the implanted device, very few precautions need be taken; it's fine to swim, surf, etc. Unfortunately, every course of antibiotics does require that a needle pierce the skin to enter the central line whose reservoir lies just beneath the skin. This needle sticking through the skin is not as stable as the Broviac or Hickman catheters. Because of the advantages of each type of device, most CF physicians and patients (or their families) who have needed permanent or semipermanent IV have felt that if they were going to require relatively short courses of IV treatment with long periods between courses, the totally implanted devices were the best, but if they were likely to be on IV's more than off, then the Broviac or Hickman catheters served them better.

Complications

Infection is the most common serious complication that can occur with a central line. As already discussed, a central line infection can be a medical emergency, and at best usually means removing the infected line and replacing it with another one. There is a limit to the number of times this can be done, because once a long line has been in a particular vein, it can be difficult to put another line back through the same vein.

A very rare complication, *air embolism,* can be fatal. This happens when the central line has been opened to the air (rather than clamping it before connecting it to the medication tubing) and the patient takes a big breath, allowing air to rush into the line, and then into the heart. A small amount of air in the line will do no harm, but a large amount can be extremely dangerous. This can be guarded against by not leaving the line open to air; older children and adults can be careful to hold their breath for the short period of time that the line might be open. The danger of air accidentally entering a central line does not exist with the Mediport or Infusaport systems, since they are not uncapped when hooked to the bottle or bag of medication.

Bleeding from accidentally uncapping the central line can be serious, since the tip of the line is in an area of very high blood flow.

Fortunately, most of these complications are quite uncommon when central lines are taken good care of.

Nutritional Treatment Aids

Some patients who need nutritional supplements can be helped by special procedures and devices (see Chapter 4). These may include central lines for the administration of high calorie intravenous feeding, the so-called "hyperalimentation" solutions. The procedures, care, and risks for central lines used for hyperalimentation are the same as those used for antibiotics.

Extra calories can also be given through the normal digestive tract, with three different types of tube feedings.

Nasogastric Tubes

"NG tubes" go through the nose (*naso-*) and pass down the throat into the stomach (*gastric*). If a thin tube is passed this way just before bedtime, a person can sleep while high calorie formula is slowly pumped through it overnight. As discussed in Chapter 4, this method of feeding has been successful for a number of people with CF. It has the disadvantage of having to insert the tube through the nose and swallow it each night and remove it each morning, and although this is not a painful procedure, it is uncomfortable. A great advantage of this method of tube feeding compared with the two other methods (discussed below) is that the tube is out during the day.

Gastrostomy

A gastrostomy tube ("G-tube") passes directly into the stomach through a hole made in the abdominal wall by a surgeon. This tube is very safe, and provides a direct route for high calorie formulas to be fed (usually at night, while the patient sleeps). There are several disadvantages: (1) It requires a surgical procedure, usually with general anesthesia, and makes the patient quite sore for the first few days after the procedure. (2) The tube is always present, even during the day when it's not being used. (The reason it must be there even when it's not being used is that the hole would close, and heal shut within hours if the tube weren't there to keep it open.) Having the tube in is not uncomfortable, but many people don't feel comfortable wearing a bathing suit if they have a tube sticking out of their abdomen. (A device called a "button" is available which has solved this problem: it is a very short tube that can go in the stoma and keep it open, but while barely extending beyond the skin. It can easily be covered with a small Band-Aid (3).) If someone has a tendency toward gastroesophageal reflux (see Chapter 2), filling the stomach during sleep may worsen that problem.

However, the advantages are also considerable: (1) It works: This method has been very successful for a large number of CF patients. (2) It avoids the discomfort of passing a nasogastric tube each evening and morning. (3) If the tube falls out, it can just be put back in (if it's replaced within a few hours). (4) It does not interfere with any activities (except for the embarrassment); it is safe to go swimming or play any sports with it in place. (5) If and when you get to a point where you no longer want or need to use it, it can simply be taken out.

Jejunostomy

The "J-tube" is very similar to the gastrostomy tube, except that the surgical opening is made in the jejunum (the second part of the small intestine) rather than in the stomach. It has one main advantage over the gastrostomy tube, mainly, that it avoids the problem of gastroesophageal reflux. Since the formula doesn't go into the stomach, it can't back up into the esophagus. A minor advantage is that the tube used is smaller than most gastrostomy tubes, and therefore is more readily coiled up flat against the abdomen out of the way.

There are several disadvantages to the J-tube: (1) Placing it initially is more difficult than placing the G-tube. (2) If the tube falls out, it is somewhat more difficult to replace than the G-tube, especially if it falls out within the first weeks after it's been placed. Replacing it may even require another operation. Once it's been in for a few weeks or months, though, a track is well-established and if the tube falls out or gets pulled out accidentally, it can be replaced readily by just putting it back in (no surgery is necessary).

Complications of Gastrostomy and Jejunostomy Tubes

Both kinds of tubes are relatively trouble-free, but some complications can occur. The first isn't really a complication, since it is to be expected, namely, the discomfort for the first few days after they are placed. Any surgery on the abdomen will make someone uncomfortable, perhaps very uncomfortable, for a few days and placing these tubes is no exception. Occasionally, the tubes may leak, especially when someone coughs. In most circumstances, the leaking can be taken care of by pulling the tube more tightly against the abdominal wall. Some people may develop tender scar (*granulation*) tissue at the site of the stoma. This can be removed painlessly in the surgeon's office.

Oxygen-Delivery Systems

In most patients who need oxygen, the simplest way to deliver the oxygen to the patient is through nasal cannulas (this is discussed more fully in *Appendix B: Medications*). However, there is one relatively new method which fits in the category of this chapter, namely *transtracheal oxygen delivery*. This method involves the placement of a tiny tracheostomy (a hole in the neck that goes into the trachea), through which a small plastic tube can be inserted. In turn, this tube can be connected to the oxygen tubing. The procedure can be performed in a physician's office and doesn't require general anesthesia. The advantages of this method of getting oxygen are cosmetic and financial. The cosmetic advantage is that the oxygen tubing can go under the clothes, and a scarf or turtleneck can cover the tracheostomy. (With nasal cannulas, the oxygen tubing wraps around the head.) The financial advantage is that much less oxygen is needed if it is fed directly into the trachea than if it goes through the nose. A fair number of adults with emphysema have used this method to good advantage, and a few people with CF have also used this method for getting extra oxygen. If you find yourself in the position of needing oxygen, it may be worth discussing with your physician.

6/ Daily Life

David M. Orenstein and Denise R. Rodgers

There are many aspects of daily life that are altered very little by having cystic fibrosis (CF): babies cry and laugh, and children still sleep through the night, wake up, go to the bathroom, have breakfast, go to school, play with friends, play sports, do homework and chores, watch TV, and go to parties. They may go on trips with or without their families. They grow up and finish school; they take jobs; many marry, and may decide to raise a family. It is very important for a child's emotional well-being, and that of the family, that daily life be approached with these expectations. The emotional aspect of living with CF is discussed in Chapter 9, and the issues that relate specifically to adults are addressed in Chapter 10. This chapter addresses the few areas in which CF does have an effect on the patient's (or family's) daily life.

In most stages of life, having CF requires some form of chest physical therapy, anywhere from one to four times a day. Approximately 90 percent of people with CF must remember, or be reminded, to take digestive enzymes with each meal and usually with snacks. Most patients will also have to take vitamins each day, and many will need to take antibiotics by mouth fairly frequently.

Clinic visits for checkups will be required anywhere from one to eight times a year, depending on your physician's approach and your health. These visits are very important for health maintenance (see Chapter 1, *Steps Toward Treating Worsened Lungs*).

During periods of pulmonary exacerbation (see Chapter 1), it may be necessary to come into the hospital for 1–3 weeks, or to receive IV antibiotics at home (see Chapter 5). This treatment may be necessary for as many as one in every four patients, and for one to three times each year.

Patients who have more severe lung disease may need to adjust the intensity of their physical exertion, and a very few may even need to wear oxygen while they are up and around and perhaps during sleep, but this is a very small proportion of patients.

Mealtimes should not be too different for people with CF than it would be if they didn't have CF, except for remembering to take the enzymes. If someone has had trouble putting (or keeping) weight on, there may be meals with added fats and calories to help with growth (see Chapter 4).

MEDICATIONS AND TREATMENTS: WHO'S IN CHARGE?

During a child's early years, the parents are responsible for the medication and must know which medicines should be taken when, why they are needed, and what additional treatments are required. By the time a young adult leaves home, he or she must be in charge of these areas. Most experts feel that a good time for the transition in this responsibility from the parents to the young patient is early in the teenage years. This period is both a good and a bad time for accomplishing this end. It is a good time because the teenager is wanting very much to become independent of the parent, and is looking for ways to assert that independence. Teenagers welcome the trust that accompanies responsibility as well as the absence of nagging that results when they have learned all their medications and take them faithfully.

Adolescence can be a difficult time, however, for the transition in responsibility, because in normal teenage rebellion against authority there is a strong urge to ignore what the parents want. When the teenager has CF, what the parents want is for the teenager to take the prescribed medications and treatments in order to stay well. This may be an area where the teenager is able to exert some control, and the relatively common feeling of invulnerability ("nothing will happen to me") may just add to the appeal of not taking medications. As with so many other aspects of the teenager's life, the best solution is to encourage him or her to take full responsibility for medications and treatments, but to be aware of what is and is not being done, and to encourage the best cooperation possible. To encourage this self-care and independence, the physician may choose to meet with the patient alone, and to have the parents sit in the waiting room during clinic visits.

DAYCARE

Daycare has become very common for many families with babies, especially if both parents work. Babies in daycare get more colds than babies kept at home. Babies with CF will get neither more nor fewer colds than the other babies, but some of these colds may develop into bronchial infections (pulmonary exacerbations). This fact has made some families try to avoid daycare. For the first months of an infant's life, when the bronchi are very tiny and when infants with CF may have more trouble keeping the bronchi clear, it may be advisable to delay daycare. However, if this is financially difficult, it should not be considered a major setback. Remember that the goal of avoiding all colds is impossible to achieve, especially if there are other children in the family, and that careful attention to an infant's health, with quick treatment for any pulmonary infections, is likely to result in very good maintenance of health.

Occasionally, a misguided daycare supervisor, parent, or even physician may be concerned that the presence of an infant with CF will pose a danger to the other children in daycare. *Cystic fibrosis is not contagious.* Even if a baby with CF is coughing a lot, the bacteria in the lungs of someone with CF are not dangerous to children without CF. Of course, a baby with CF can get a regular cold, just like any other baby, and pass that cold on to anyone else, but babies with CF should not be excluded from daycare just because of having CF, or because of cough.

SCHOOL

School is very important for all children, and virtually all children with CF should be able to go to school and carry a full load, including homework and extracurricular activities. When a child has a lung infection, he or she may not feel as well as usual, but in most cases this should not interfere with education. Children should be encouraged to go to school, even if they are coughing more than their usual, as long as they are receiving the appropriate treatment (antibiotics, and increased chest physical therapy treatments).

Teachers may need to be educated about CF (the CF Foundation has a very good little booklet designed for teachers) to make a very few special considerations for the child with CF. They need to be aware that the child with CF is likely to have more cough than other children, and should never be discouraged from coughing. The child with CF may also need to have more frequent bathroom privileges.

Homework should be required from the child with CF, just as from his or her peers. There should be almost no exceptions to this rule. Even if a child has to be hospitalized, he or she should keep up with school work. If a child is hospitalized, the school district should provide tutoring to enable the child to keep up with the class.

Gym class is as important (or even more important) for children with CF as for other children. Physical education class should not be graded on the basis of athletic performance for any child, especially those who might have a physical reason for lower than normal performance, as a child with CF and lung disease might have.

SPORTS AND EXERCISE

In general, there is no reason for children, adolescents, and adults with CF to avoid exercise. Exercise is good for most people, including people with CF. Everyone, with CF or without it, needs to adjust the amount and intensity of exercise to his or her own abilities and needs, but this can be done fairly easily. (Exercise and sports are discussed more in Chapter 7.)

VISITS WITH FRIENDS

Visiting with friends, either at their house or your own is an important part of growing up, learning to get along with others, and learning to become independent away from home. Children and adolescents with CF should have these same opportunities as anyone else. In most cases, special arrangements will have to be made to be certain that medications are being taken and that treatments are being done. In some cases, for a single overnighter for a grade-school child, it might not be a problem to skip a single day's treatment, but this should not become a habit. Adolescents who give themselves their own treatments should be able to do this anywhere. If either part of the visiting pair is sick, changes may have to be made, but this is no different from what would be done if neither child had CF.

SMOKING

People with any form of lung disease should not smoke, nor should they inhale other people's smoke. This is certainly true for people with CF. Smoke is harmful to children's lungs, even if the lungs are normal. Someone who has abnormal lungs, especially if asthma is part of the condition, has a greatly increased risk of complications if he or she must breathe cigarette smoke. Smoke from cigarettes can be harmful to a child's lungs even if the person smoking the cigarette loves the child very much. Parents whose child has CF should stop smoking immediately, and smoking should not be allowed in their home. Most people, including smokers, know that smoking is very harmful to the smoker; not everyone realizes that it is also harmful to the lungs of children who are forced to breathe in the second-hand smoke.

Many parents who have been unsuccessful at stopping smoking are able to stop when they realize that it is not just for their own health but for the children's as well. If you cannot stop right away, it is essential that you stop smoking in the house. If you're smoking in the same house, the baby will get the fumes. You must especially never smoke in the car, since that is an enclosed space where smoke can get very thick and irritating. If you need help stopping, your physician may be able to help. For someone who is truly addicted to cigarettes, the addiction is every bit as serious as—and harder to break than—a heroin addiction. Nicotine chewing gum has been helpful for people who are dedicated to stopping smoking but can't do it on their own.

TRAVEL

Patients with CF can travel, just as people without CF can. There are a few practical considerations for the traveling CF patient.

Remember to bring your medicines Some medications used for CF patients (especially enzymes) may not be carried in just any pharmacy, so it may be difficult to replace medications while you're away from your regular drug store. If you travel out of state, you may find that a pharmacy won't accept your doctor's prescription if he or she is not licensed in the state you're visiting. In most cases, pharmacists are very helpful, and will do what they can to provide you with the service you need, but it's better to be prepared for a problem.

Remember to bring any equipment you might need for aerosols or postural drainage treatments If you're traveling to a different country, you may need to bring special electrical outlet adaptors for whatever electrical equipment you use, since different countries use different power sources. Adaptors are available to enable you to convert the power source to fit your own equipment.

High altitude If you live at or near sea level and travel to higher altitudes, you may experience difficulty because of the lower oxygen pressures at altitude. The air in Denver, for example, has only 80 percent as much oxygen as that in San Diego or Boston. Someone whose lungs are in excellent condition should have no trouble in these places, but someone who has serious lung involvement may be comfortable and safe at sea level, but develop problems in the mountains. It is a good idea to discuss travel plans with your doctor before going.

Airplane travel Commercial airlines pressurize their cabins to 5000–8000 feet. That means that the oxygen level inside the cabin is comparable to Denver's or a place even higher. Once again, if you need oxygen at sea level, you will need more in an airplane, and if you are close to needing it at home, you may need it while you fly. The major airlines are used to dealing with requests for oxygen during flights, and usually are very helpful, *but most insist that you contact them well in advance* to let them know about your plans and needs (usually there is a special medical department to contact at the airline).

SUMMER CAMP

Summer camps can provide valuable experience for children and adolescents, and most children and adolescents with CF should be able to attend camp if they want to. Most children whose lungs are in good shape and whose digestion is fairly well controlled with enzymes should be able to attend any kind of camp, as long as arrangements for medications and treatments can be made with the camp physicians and nurses. Many areas have CF camps, which have some special advantages and disadvantages. The advantages of CF camp include staff who are familiar with CF and who are equipped to give regular treatments, and the opportunity for children to get to know other children with CF and share their experiences and feelings, which increase their understanding of their condition. The main disadvantage, especially for someone who is quite healthy, is the danger of limiting a child's world to the CF world.

WHERE TO LIVE

People often wonder if there are areas of the country that are better than others for children (and adults) with CF. From what is known now, the answer is no. In individual patients, it is possible that they might do better in one geographic location than another, but so many factors influence how someone will do, and patients are so different from each other, that no one place has the perfect combination of factors that make for good health for all people with CF.

Cities and states differ in the amount of pollution, cold, wetness, and allergens, and in the availability of good medical care. While one might think that the cold, wet, polluted, industrial, northeastern cities (Cleveland, Pittsburgh, Boston, Toronto, etc.) would be the worst places for CF patients to live, national survival statistics, which measure how long people live, show that it is exactly these cities which have the *best* CF survival. The explanation almost certainly lies in the fact that these cities have had excellent CF centers for the longest time. Excellent CF centers now exist in most regions of the United States, Canada, Europe, and Australia, and most likely, in 10 years or so, the survival statistics will begin to reflect this change. Most CF physicians feel that ready access to a good CF center is important, but other than this criterion, there is very little basis for recommending one geographic area over another for someone with CF.

7 Exercise

David M. Orenstein

Everyone is interested in exercise these days. People with cystic fibrosis (CF) are no exception. Exercise done properly, in the right amount, the right intensity, and with the proper safety precautions, can be fun and beneficial for nearly everyone. Again, people with CF are no exception.

EFFECTS OF EXERCISE ON PEOPLE WITHOUT CYSTIC FIBROSIS

Single Sessions of Exercise

When someone begins muscular exercise, the body has to make some fast adaptations, most of which relate to supplying the exercising muscles with considerably more oxygen than is needed at rest. These adaptations help the muscles remove excess carbon dioxide which is produced when they are active. Muscles are able to contract and move the body *without* oxygen, but this is much more difficult than muscular work performed *with* adequate oxygen. Work that is performed without adequate oxygen being supplied to the muscles is called *anaerobic* work; work that is performed with enough oxygen is called *aerobic* work. Anaerobic exercise can only be carried out for a period of seconds or minutes, whereas aerobic exercise can be sustained for many minutes or even hours. Anaerobic exercise is not only more difficult and less efficient than aerobic exercise but also results in the production of lactic acid in the muscles, and in the production of considerably more carbon dioxide, which then has to be removed.

Since oxygen is supplied to the exercising muscles (and carbon dioxide is removed) by circulating blood, one of the first changes at the beginning of exercise is an increase in blood flow to the active muscle. Since the heart has to pump more blood, it has to pump faster, and the heart rate (pulse) increases. The heart rate reaches a maximum which can be predicted accurately from the person's age: maximum heart rate = 220 − age (in years).

Thus, a 20-year-old person would have a predicted maximum heart rate of
220 − 20 = 200 beats per minute. It is also necessary to increase the amount
of oxygen available to the blood, and, especially with anaerobic exercise, to
increase the disposal of carbon dioxide. The increase in oxygen supply and
carbon dioxide removal are both accomplished by increasing the amount of
air that is breathed each minute. The accuracy of these adjustments is astounding, as you've already seen in Chapter 1. During heavy exercise, the
heart may increase its output five- or sixfold, and the lungs may bring in
(and exhale) five to 10 times as much air as they do during naps, and yet,
the level of oxygen and carbon dioxide in the bloodstream remains nearly
constant.

It takes anywhere from a few seconds to 1½ minutes to adjust the amount
of blood the heart pumps to the exercising muscles. Therefore, during the
first seconds of exercise, the muscles are undersupplied with oxygen. In
other words, the first seconds of any form of exercise are anaerobic exercise.
Exercise that is strictly "stop-and-go," in which you exercise, rest, then
exercise again (for example, racquet sports) is anaerobic exercise. Exercise
is also anaerobic if it is very heavy work and the muscles demand more
oxygen than can be supplied (for example, heavy weight lifting, running, or
riding a bike up a steep hill). In contrast, aerobic exercise is a low intensity,
rhythmic type of activity, such as walking, swimming, easy jogging, and bike
riding.

Exercise in the Heat

The more someone exercises, especially in hot weather, the more heat the
body produces. If the body temperature becomes too high it can be dangerous, so there has to be a way for body temperature to remain relatively
constant. This is accomplished through several mechanisms. The first is that
a greater amount of blood than usual is sent to the skin, especially the scalp
and hands. This is a way of bringing the warmth of the body close to the
surface, where it can be given off to the surrounding air (unless the air is
hotter than body temperature). If all of the blood stayed in the heart and
other internal organs, it would be insulated by the skin, muscles, and fat and
the heat would build up. The other way of giving off excess heat is through
sweating. As sweat evaporates, it cools the surface of the body. This is why
you sweat when you exercise, especially in the heat.

Exercise Tolerance

When someone is given a test on an exercise cycle, it becomes progressively more difficult to pedal and, eventually, *everyone* will get to the point
where he or she can no longer pedal. In most healthy people, the point at

which this occurs is determined by two factors. The first is that the heart reaches a point at which it can no longer increase the amount of blood it pumps to the muscles, so the muscles become relatively undersupplied with blood and oxygen and fatigued. This usually happens when the heart rate has reached the maximum limit. If a 20-year-old person is exercising so hard that the heart rate is 200 beats per minute, it will not be able to go much faster, so the amount of blood being pumped out will not be able to increase any further.

The second limiting factor may be the muscles themselves: there is a limit to how much oxygen the muscles can process, so they may become fatigued even though enough oxygen has been delivered. In someone with normal lungs, the lungs are never the limiting factor in exercise. Even at total exhaustion, the lungs have considerable reserve. Recall from Chapter 1 that the maximum voluntary ventilation (MVV) is the measurement of the largest amount of air someone can move in and out of the lungs in a minute. During exercise, even at the point of total exhaustion, most people don't use any more than 70 percent of their MVV; that is, their lungs could still deliver another 30 percent effort. But this wouldn't help, since other factors would have impeded the exercise before the extra breathing reserves were needed.

Repeated Sessions of Exercise (Exercise Programs)

If you exercise each day, or at least 3 days a week, for a certain minimum amount (10–30 minutes a day), and at a certain minimum intensity (hard enough to raise your heart rate to approximately 75 percent of its maximum, which is around 150 beats per minute for adolescents and young adults), after a few weeks (6–12 weeks), you will become more fit, that is, you will be able to do more of the same kind of exercise with less stress on your body. If the type of exercise you were doing each day was aerobic, then you will increase your *aerobic fitness*. If it was anaerobic exercise, then your anaerobic fitness will increase. Jogging 30 minutes each day will make it much easier for you to jog, but it will not make you able to lift 200 pounds, whereas lifting weights every day may make your muscles stronger (and bigger) for weight-lifting tasks, but will not improve your endurance or your ability to carry out prolonged walks or bike rides.

With repeated aerobic exercise sessions, involving walking or jogging, one of the ways in which you become more fit is that your heart is able to pump more blood *with each beat,* and therefore you need fewer heart beats to deliver the same amount of blood to the muscles. You can see this change by checking your heart rate for a certain work load before you start an exercise program, then rechecking it after a few months of exercise. The easiest "work load" to check is no work at all, that is, measure your resting heart rate. The more fit someone is, the lower his or her resting heart rate.

You may know runners who brag about having a resting heart rate of 45 or 50 beats per minute.

Another change that occurs with a training program and increased fitness is in the muscles themselves: They become able to process much more oxygen and to put that oxygen to use in performing work.

One change that *does not* occur with an exercise training program is in lung function. Most scientific studies have shown no important changes in lung function in healthy people after they train and become very fit. Since lung function doesn't have much to do with one's exercise ability if the lungs are normal, this doesn't make much difference to most people.

Heat Training

Another change that comes with an exercise program, especially if it's been carried out in the heat, is that you become heat acclimatized, that is, you can withstand exercise and heat stress better than you could before you got in shape. Several changes account for this improved heat tolerance. The first is just that exercise itself is easier because of being more fit (lower heart rate, etc.), without regard to the heat. But additional changes occur that are related specifically to increased heat tolerance. People who train in the heat begin to sweat earlier during an exercise session, thus cooling themselves earlier through evaporation. In addition, and quite remarkably, when someone without CF trains in the heat for several weeks, the sweat that is produced contains less salt. This may be the body's way of preserving salt, since much salt can be lost when someone sweats excessively. (People running a marathon can easily lose 5–10 pounds of sweat in 3 or 4 hours.)

EFFECTS OF EXERCISE IN PEOPLE WITH CYSTIC FIBROSIS

Single Sessions of Exercise

The responses to exercise in people with CF are generally similar to those of people who don't have CF. To meet the increased oxygen needs of exercising muscles and to remove carbon dioxide, both the heart's output and the amount of breathing are considerably increased. If the person's lung function is normal or nearly normal, he or she will have exactly the same responses to exercise as anyone else. However, there are some differences in the response to exercise in someone with CF whose pulmonary function is not normal. One difference is that people with CF frequently stop exercising before their rate has reached the maximum predicted based upon age. In these cases, the minute ventilation (the amount of air being breathed each minute) may be very large in comparison with the person's capacity or reserve. Remember that people with normal lungs seldom breathe more than

70 percent of their MVV, even during strenuous exercise. People with CF often use more than 80 percent of their MVV (in some cases, more than 100 percent of their "maximum" capacity is used). Even as you can't expect a person with a normal heart to make the heart beat faster than its maximum, you can't expect *anyone*—with or without healthy lungs—to be able to use more than 100% of the lungs' capacity.

Most patients with CF maintain their blood levels of oxygen and carbon dioxide during exercise. In some patients, the blood oxygen level actually *increases* with exercise. However, in people with severe lung disease, the blood oxygen level may fall during exercise, and in some of these patients, the carbon dioxide level may increase. [This decrease in oxygen level does not occur in anyone whose forced expired volume (FEV_1) is greater than 50 percent of their forced vital capacity (FVC; see Chapter 1), and it doesn't occur in most people whose FEV_1 is that low.] This means that for the amount of oxygen being used and the amount of carbon dioxide being produced by the exercising muscles, the person is not breathing enough. It is not known if this is harmful, but most CF physicians recommend that patients avoid this situation. That does not mean to avoid exercise altogether. Specific exercise guidelines are discussed later in this chapter.

Many people with CF will cough during or after exercise. This may be distressing to someone who is watching, if they don't know about CF, and may be somewhat uncomfortable to the person coughing, but it is not dangerous. In fact, it is probably helpful in bringing mucus up out of the lungs.

Exercise in the Heat

Having CF should not prevent someone from exercising in the heat. People with CF have the same ability as people without CF to keep their body temperature down while exercising in hot weather. However, since they have the same mechanisms for doing this, including sweating, and since CF sweat is so much saltier than any other sweat, athletes with CF lose much more salt than their non-CF friends. They may lose so much that the blood levels of sodium and chloride drop. In most cases this does not cause a problem. Young people with CF also have an extremely accurate salt "thermostat" that enables them to know exactly how much salt they need to take to replace what they've lost. Replacing salt is something that can be done over a period of hours, and does not have to be done immediately after it's lost.

Replacing lost fluid is quite another matter, though, for anyone, with or without CF. It is very important for all people who exercise in the heat to drink plenty of fluid, but it is particularly important for children and adults with CF to drink while they exercise in hot weather, because while their salt "thermostat" works very well, their fluid "thermostat" is a little sluggish.

All children tend to drink less fluid than they lose during exercise in the heat, but children with CF are especially neglectful of drinking as much as they need.

Exercise Tolerance

Many children and adults with CF who have good lung function are limited in their exercise capacity by the same factors that limit their classmates; namely, the heart reaches a limit to how much blood it can pump, and/or the muscles reach a limit to how much oxygen they can process. These factors will be especially limiting if someone has not exercised much and is out of shape. But those whose lungs are affected more extensively by their CF are likely to be limited by the lungs before the heart and muscles are pushed to their limits. This does not necessarily mean that their blood oxygen levels will fall, but rather that the work of breathing may just become too great and they will need to stop because of that discomfort. Even in most people whose oxygen level does fall, it is probably the discomfort of hard breathing and not the lowered oxygen level which forces them to stop running or pedalling. There are certainly a few people who benefit from using oxygen during exercise, and are able to do considerably more exercise if they use extra oxygen when they are active.

Although coughing may be severe, it seldom limits exercise.

Exercise Programs for People with Cystic Fibrosis

Exercise programs have the same benefit for people with CF that they have for people without CF, namely, increasing fitness. "Increased fitness" is defined as being able to do more physical work, and having a lower heart rate for the same work load. Some studies have shown better lung function after a CF exercise training program, and other studies have shown no change in lung function. For people with normal lungs, strenuous aerobic exercise programs should raise the heart rate to 75 percent of its maximum, or about 150 beats per minute. Many people with CF will not be able to exercise this hard, because their breathing will stop them before their heart rate has gotten that high. This does not mean that someone with CF cannot become more fit. In fact, it seems that CF patients can become more fit by exercising hard enough to raise their heart rates to 75 percent of their own maximum, and not the maximum that you'd predict on the basis of their age. Thus, if someone with CF has a maximum heart rate of 150 beats per minute (that is, the pulse goes up to 150 during the most strenuous exercise which he or she can tolerate), that person will be able to benefit from regular exercise sessions with the heart beating around 115 beats a minute (roughly 75 percent of 150).

Fortunately, it's not necessary to measure the heart rate precisely during all exercise sessions to know if you're working hard enough to bring about improvements; instead, you can strive for a pleasantly tired feeling. If you're not at all tired, you are not working hard enough. On the other hand, if you're so tired that you don't feel at all good, you're pushing yourself harder than you need. That becomes important in planning a long-term exercise program, because human nature is such that no one wants to do unpleasant things, and exercise is no exception: if your exercise sessions leave you exhausted and feeling bad, you will be much more likely to find excuses to skip them than if they are enjoyable. In the section after next there will be an introduction to the nitty-gritty of carrying out an exercise program.

Heat Training in Cystic Fibrosis

Like everyone else, *people with CF can become adapted to exercise in the heat.* If you exercise in the heat every day for a week or more, at the end of that period, your heart rate and body temperature will be lower when you exercise than they were at the beginning.

When you have CF, you are likely to lose large amounts of sodium and chloride during each exercise session in the heat. If you allow yourself to eat and drink without restriction, you will find that you automatically select items that will completely replace the lost salt. This is very important, because a major difference between the normal response to heat training and the CF response is that CF sweat glands cannot decrease the salt content of sweat. This means that even though you have greater tolerance for exercise and heat stress, you still lose much more salt than is normal. In addition, after you've trained for a while, you will begin to sweat earlier in the exercise session (this change occurs in *everyone* during heat training) and you will also be able to exercise for a longer period, thus losing even more salt after you've become adapted to the heat.

GUIDELINES FOR AN EXERCISE PROGRAM

General

Medical Advice

Check with your doctor before you start. If your lungs are severely affected by CF, your doctor may recommend an exercise test first to check your oxygen level. If your FEV_1 is less than 50 percent of your FVC, it's a particularly good idea to see if your oxygen level falls during exercise, and if so, at what intensity: If your oxygen level is good until your heart rate reaches 150 beats per minute, it's relatively easy to keep your exercise program light enough that your heart rate stays below 145. Your doctor might even want to prescribe some oxygen for you to use while you exercise. For most people with CF, this will not be necessary.

Time Allotment

Set aside a time to exercise. This should amount to about 30 minutes a day, three to five times a week for the exercise itself, plus whatever time you need to shower and dress. You should guard this exercise time jealously and keep it for yourself. It doesn't matter what time of day you exercise. Some people prefer to exercise in the morning, whereas others prefer to wait until they've been awake and active for several hours. Of course, if your exercise is in gym class or with a team, you won't have much choice as to timing.

Type of Activity

Pick an activity that is a good aerobic conditioner. These activities are ones which are continuous, not stop-and-go; they are light enough that they can be carried out for many minutes at a time, without causing total exhaustion. Typical aerobic activities that are discussed below in greater detail include running, swimming, and biking. Others include rowing, skating, cross-country skiing, and vigorous walking.

Activities that are *an*aerobic include weight training, most racquet sports, and volleyball. There is nothing wrong with these activities, and many are fun; some may even make you stronger and build your muscles, but they will probably not help your endurance. Boxing is too dangerous even to be mentioned as an activity, except to condemn it.

Regular daily activities should not be overlooked in planning a more active lifestyle. If you usually walk the dog around a short block, try going around a long block instead; walk or ride a bike to the corner store when you run out of milk instead of getting a ride; take the stairs instead of the elevator whenever possible; and so on. Try cutting down on TV time in favor of exercising time. It does you a lot more good to walk or run around the block than to watch someone else doing it on TV.

PACING YOURSELF

Getting going. Whatever activity you pick, remember not to overdo it, especially when you first begin to train. Listen carefully to what your body is telling you about how hard or fast or far you're going. It's much better to take a few days, weeks, or even months to work your way up to the desired amount of exercise than to get injured or discouraged by trying too much too soon. If you haven't been particularly active, limit your first exercise session to no more than 10 minutes. Continue to exercise for 10 minutes each day for the first week. With each successive week, try adding 2 minutes to each session. By the time several months have passed, you'll find that you're exercising for as long as 30 minutes.

Listen to your body: If you're getting winded, go slower until you've caught your breath, and then continue at an easier pace. If you feel as though you've hardly exerted yourself after 10 minutes, you can push a little harder for a little longer.

Injuries

Minor injuries can occur with most forms of exercise. Don't ignore them. While you can continue to exercise with some discomfort, real pain is a signal to stop. Let a few days pass without exercising, and if your pain persists, inform your doctor.

Medications, Food, and Drink

If you have asthma or if you take any inhaled bronchodilators, it's advisable to take an inhalation before you exercise. It is not wise to exercise after a heavy meal; in fact, waiting several hours after a meal before you run or swim will make your exercise more pleasant. If you're exercising in warm weather, you should drink while you exercise—probably even more than you think you need. You do not need to take salt pills.

Running

Equipment

The only special equipment you need for running is a good pair of running shoes. Gym shoes or tennis shoes are not appropriate for regular running. A long-term running program involves a lot of pounding of your feet on the pavement. If you don't have the proper shoes, this pounding travels from your feet to your shins, knees, and hips and can cause an injury. It is advisable to buy your shoes in a store that specializes in runners' supplies. When shopping for running shoes, pick a shoe that feels good on your foot. Do not expect an uncomfortable shoe to "break in" after a while the way a leather shoe might (most running shoes are made of synthetic materials which do not change their shape with time and wear).

Clothes

You can run in clothes that you probably already have. For summer running, dress as lightly as possible. Nylon shorts and shirts are light and dry out quickly, but cotton is more absorbent. For running in colder weather, you are more likely to overdress than underdress. When the temperature is below freezing, cotton socks and sweat-pants or stretch tights are the best. Cover your chest with several light layers rather than one heavy layer. On the coldest days, a T-shirt, cotton turtleneck, and hooded cotton sweatshirt should be enough. If it is very windy, a thin nylon shell suit over your running clothes will insulate you and keep the wind out. Be sure to cover your head with a wool cap or the hood from your sweatshirt because much of the body's heat is lost from the head. A scarf or mask over your nose and mouth may make breathing easier. Your feet are working hard, so they won't get very cold, but your hands will. To keep your hands warm, mittens or socks are better than gloves, since they let your fingers keep each other warm. Some petroleum jelly on your lips and cheeks will reduce the sting of the cold.

Starting to Run

Remember not to push yourself too hard, especially at first. You should be exercising to make yourself feel good; if you push so hard that you feel bad, you've missed the point. Start with a 10-minute run/walk session. Run slowly, and when you get tired, start walking. When you are ready, run again. Continue this for three or four sessions during your first week, trying to run for most of the 10 minutes. As the weeks go by, you should gradually add time to your run/walk sessions. Add 2 or 3 minutes each week, so that, after 7–10 weeks, you are running for most of each 30-minute session. If it takes longer to add the extra minutes, don't worry, there's no rush. It doesn't matter how far you go or how long it takes you to work up to 30 minutes of running.

Safety

You should be able to avoid injury to your muscles if you warm up properly before running, stretch and cool down afterwards, and build up gradually to a regular exercise program. However, if you feel pain after running, be sure to have it checked. Other safety factors to consider include not running in traffic or other polluted areas, and not running in dark clothes at night. You can avoid these problems by running on an athletic field, golf course, track, or jogging trail rather than on the sidewalk or street.

If you start your running program in the spring, summer, or fall, you may become discouraged when the weather turns bad in the winter months. There is really no reason you shouldn't run in the winter, as long as you dress properly. Running on icy or slippery surfaces is dangerous, so be careful and sensible about running in the winter; a broken leg or sprained ankle will not promote your general conditioning.

Swimming

Where to Swim

You will need a pool, lake, river, or ocean. Unless you live in a part of the country where the weather is good and you can swim outside all year round, you will want to swim in a pool that is convenient to get to and affordable to use. A summer swimming program at a beach or lake won't give you any long-term benefit if you only swim for 2 or 3 months out of the year. Additionally, rivers and oceans have currents, waves, and tides that may interfere with a regular, sustained swimming program. If you don't have a pool or ocean in your backyard, there are a lot of places where you should be able to swim for free or at a moderate cost. Many high schools and colleges have pools that are open to the public during certain hours. Many people swim at municipal or community pools. Most YMCAs and many health clubs and hotels have swimming pools that can be joined for a reasonable fee.

Equipment

Once you have found a place to swim, the only equipment or special clothing you will really need is a bathing suit. For a regular exercise program, a one-piece nylon tank suit is best. A nylon suit will wear well and dry out quickly. Goggles are useful if you are swimming in a pool or in salt water, since both chlorine and salt can be very irritating to the eyes. If you wear glasses or contact lenses you can purchase goggles with corrective lenses for very reasonable cost (ask your eye doctor for details). If you have long hair, a bathing cap will keep your hair out of your face, as well as out of a pool's filter system.

Safety

NEVER SWIM ALONE! There should always be a lifeguard at the pool or beach. While you are probably less likely to drown in a swimming pool than in a lake, river, or ocean, always make sure that there is a lifeguard present. Failing that, use the "buddy system," swimming with a friend who can pull you out of the water or run for help if you need it. You should also learn some basic water safety techniques. The risk of pulling muscles or tendons while swimming is much less than while running or bicycling. If you are swimming smoothly, your muscles should get an even workout. Most injuries occur from diving into shallow water, swimming into the side of the pool, or sustaining cuts from rocks or trash on the bottom of a river or lake.

Learning to Swim

Swimming is most enjoyable when you have a smooth, comfortable stroke. If you do not know how to swim well or if you want to improve your stroke, swimming lessons will be helpful. This does not mean that you have to start training to make the Olympic team, but you should be able to execute the various strokes properly. As in running and bicycling, the goal is not speed, but rather sustained, even exercise over time. There are many places where you can learn to swim. The Red Cross and the YMCA are probably best known for their swimming programs, but any reputable class will do. Many places offer swimming lessons designed especially for adults.

Starting to Swim

As with running, don't push yourself too hard or too fast at first. A 10-minute session that alternates a strenuous stroke like the crawl (free-style) with a more restful stroke (breaststroke or sidestroke) should get you off to a good start. Try to schedule your swimming sessions three or four times each week for the first few weeks. Gradually work up to longer sessions by adding a few minutes to each session after the first week or two. Your goal should be to swim for at least 30 minutes during each session. Again, remember that you can take as many weeks as you need to reach this goal. It doesn't matter how many laps you swim or how fast you swim them.

Bicycling

Equipment

If you plan to cycle out-of-doors, a sturdy bike with 3 to 12 speeds is your basic piece of equipment. A cycling helmet is also essential to prevent head injuries if you fall or are thrown from your bike. If you plan to cycle indoors, there are many good models of stationary exercise bikes. However, before you buy one, remember that riding a stationary bike can be extremely boring. Some people set the bike up in front of the TV and pedal as they watch. Others listen to music or read while they ride. Most people who just cycle in a bare cellar don't stay with it very long.

Preparing Your Bicycle

Your bicycle should be in good condition each time you begin a ride. Make sure that the seat is properly adjusted, because this will increase the efficiency and comfort with which you ride. Raise or lower the saddle so that your leg is fully extended when your heel is placed on the pedal at the bottom of its cycle. This will cause your leg to be slightly bent while pedalling with the ball of your foot on the pedal. Before each ride, briefly inspect the tires, brakes, and wheels of your bike to make sure that they are in good order. If any part is not working properly, have it fixed. Proper maintenance of your bike will help to ensure safe riding.

Safety

Bike paths and lightly trafficked roads are recommended over city streets and highways. Familiarize yourself with the traffic laws regarding bicycling and obey them. If you plan to ride in the evenings, be sure that you have the proper lights and reflectors on your bike and wear light-colored clothes so that motorists and other riders can see you.

Clothes

The clothes needed for bicycling are similar to those for running, except that you will build up less heat, and give off more heat on a bike than on foot, so you'll have to dress more warmly (and with more wind protection) on the bike. Be sure that your pants legs fit snugly so that they won't get caught in the gears or chain.

Starting to Cycle

As with running and swimming, start out slowly and build up to longer periods of exercise. A 10- to 15-minute ride three or four times a week is a good way to start out, adding extra minutes to each session after the first week or two. Alternate slow, easy riding with fast, hard riding until you are riding for 30 minutes, three to five times a week. Strive toward a continuous, comfortable ride of increasing duration, rather than a ride that covers a certain distance.

8/ Genetics

David M. Orenstein

Cystic fibrosis (CF) is a genetic disorder, meaning that it is determined by the genes which a baby has inherited. There are millions of genes located on the chromosomes within each cell in the body. The genes are made of DNA, the basic determinant of our body makeup. Genes come in pairs, with one gene having come from each parent. As a mother's eggs are formed, each egg has only one set of genes, rather than the double set that exists in all the other cells in her body. Similarly, each of the father's millions of sperm has only one gene for each characteristic. When the sperm and egg unite, the fetus they develop into will have one set of genes from the mother and one from the father. The genes determine all of our physical characteristics, from the shape of our ears to the color of our hair. What makes each of us unique physically is the combination of genes that make up our cells.

Different gene combinations work in different ways. In some cases, a gene is *dominant,* meaning that it is the gene that will be expressed, regardless of what the gene is that accompanies it. The dominant gene completely determines the outcome. An example of this is the brown hair gene. If a baby gets one brown hair gene, he or she will have brown hair, regardless of what the other hair-color gene is. In other cases, each gene contributes something so that the resulting characteristic is a combination of what each would have determined by itself. An example of this is skin color. When a very dark-skinned person and a very fair person have a baby, the baby's skin is often a color that is in between the parents' skin colors. Finally, there is the *recessive* gene, which will not be noticed at all unless it is paired with an identical gene. Red hair is a recessive characteristic, so every redhead you see has gotten a red-hair gene from each parent. A baby with one red-hair gene and one brown-hair gene will have brown hair.

Cystic fibrosis is a recessive disorder, which means that a baby who gets a CF gene from only one parent will have no evidence of CF. CF occurs *only* in a person who has gotten a CF gene from each parent. It also means that parents of a child with CF have one CF gene and one non-CF gene in each of their cells. Yet there is no evidence that they carry the CF gene at all until

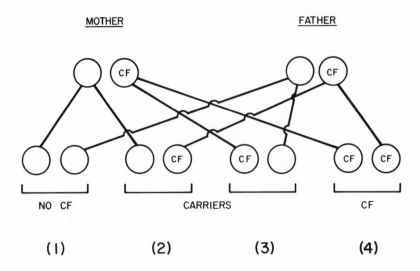

FIG. 8.1. The inheritance of CF. Each parent of a child with CF has one CF gene (*circle labelled "CF"*). The CF gene causes no problems if it is paired with a non-CF gene (*blank circle*). When two parents who carry the gene have children, each parent passes on either the CF gene or the non-CF gene. The figure shows the possible combinations of genes which children of carriers can have: **1**: A non-CF gene from both father and mother; **2**: a non-CF gene from the mother and a CF gene from the father; **3**: a CF gene from the mother and a non-CF gene from the father; or **4**: a CF gene from each parent. Each of these four combinations is just as likely to occur as the others, meaning that the chances of two carrier parents having a child with CF is one in four each time they have a child.

they have a child with CF. People who have one CF and one non-CF gene are called *carriers,* because they are not affected by the gene but carry it and can pass it along to their children. Whether their children will be affected by CF depends on what gene the other parent contributes.

Figure 8.1 shows the possible combinations if two parents who are each carriers have children. For each of them, half of their eggs or sperm will have the CF gene, and half will have the non-CF gene. The chances of a sperm that carries the CF gene fertilizing an egg with the CF gene are exactly the same as its fertilizing a non-CF egg. This means that there are only four possible combinations of genes from these parents, and each is just as likely to occur as the others. *Each time this couple has a child,* the chances are one in four that the baby will have two CF genes, and will have CF; two in four (a "fifty–fifty" chance) that the baby will have one CF gene, and therefore will not have CF but will be a carrier; and one in four that the baby will not have any CF gene at all.

Chance and statistics can be confusing to understand at first. People may assume, mistakenly, that if their chances are one in four that a baby will have CF, and they've already had a baby with CF, then the next three chil-

TABLE 8.1. *Risks of having a child with CF*

One parent	Other parent	Risk with each pregnancy
No CF history	No CF history	1 in 1600
No CF history	First cousin has CF	1 in 320
No CF history	Aunt or uncle has CF	1 in 240
No CF history	Nephew or niece has CF	1 in 160
No CF history	Sibling has CF	1 in 120
No CF history	Has CF	1 in 40
Sibling has CF	Sibling has CF	1 in 9
Sibling has CF	Has CF	1 in 3
Sibling has CF	Known carrier	1 in 6
Known carrier	Known carrier	1 in 4

dren are guaranteed not to have CF. This is not so—*each* time they have a child, there is one chance in four that the child will have CF. There are families with three children, *all* of whom have CF, and others in which both parents are carriers yet none of their children have CF. With statistical chance, the numbers work out over hundreds of thousands of cases, which doesn't much help the individual family.

Consider the example of a deck of cards. There are four suits: hearts, diamonds, spades, and clubs. If the cards are shuffled well and are not marked, and you try to pick a diamond, your chances will be one in four. But you know very well that you might pick 10 cards one time before you get a diamond, and another time you might pick four diamonds in a row. If you picked cards all morning, by the time you'd picked 1000 cards you'd have gotten pretty close to 250 diamonds, but those first few might have been almost any pattern.

Thus, while you can know the overall statistics, they won't necessarily be helpful in an individual case. Some people consider one chance in four to be great odds, while others think they're dreadful. Table 8.1 shows the chances in different situations, depending on the parents' family background.

Brothers and sisters of CF patients should all be sweat-tested to see if they have CF, even if they have been perfectly healthy, since each child born to the parents of someone with CF has a one-in-four chance of having gotten the two CF genes, and many people with CF can be healthy for a long time before symptoms appear.

CARRIERS

If a brother or sister of someone with CF does not have CF, there are two chances in three that this sibling is a carrier. As illustrated in Fig. 8.1, if both

TABLE 8.2. *Risks of being a CF carrier*

Relationship to CF patient	Risk of being a carrier
Parent of a CF patient	1 in 1 (100%)
Sibling of a CF patient	2 in 3
Aunt or uncle of CF patient	1 in 2
Nephew or niece of CF patient	1 in 3
Cousin of CF patient	1 in 4
None known	1 in 20

parents are carriers, there are only four possible combinations of CF and non-CF genes that their children could have. One combination gives CF (two CF genes); two combinations result in carriers; and one combination has no CF gene. Now once you know that a brother or sister does not have CF (and you'll know that after a properly performed sweat test), there are only three possible combinations, two of which result in carriers. Table 8.2 shows the chances of various people being CF carriers.

Until very recently there was no carrier test for CF. The only way you knew if someone was a carrier was if he or she had a child with CF. With recent advances in molecular genetics, a test is now available for family members of someone with CF that can identify carriers. At the time of the publication of this book, however, there is no test for someone who has no known family members with CF, since blood is needed from a close family member for DNA analysis (see below). It is expected that such a test will be available for everyone in the near future.

THE CYSTIC FIBROSIS GENE

Recent advances in molecular genetics have enabled researchers to zero in on the CF gene. It is now known that CF is caused by a single gene, and not a series of genes, and that it is located on the 7th of the 23 chromosomes. Its exact location on the chromosome is not yet known, but it is likely to be in the very near future. Once it is isolated, it will be possible to tell from a DNA sample from anyone whether that person is a carrier or has CF. But even without knowing its precise location, and without having isolated the gene itself, so much is known about it that by using genes that are close to the CF gene on the 7th chromosome (these are called "marker genes," or simply "markers"), very sophisticated and accurate genetic testing can be done. For nearly every couple who has had a child with CF, it is now possible to tell early in pregnancy if an expected child will have CF.

To do this testing, a sample of the amniotic fluid (the fluid that surrounds the fetus inside the uterus) must be taken by putting a needle directly through the mother's abdominal wall into the uterus (amniocentesis). This procedure has some risks, but has been used safely for many years for a range of prenatal tests, the most well known of which is the test for Down's Syndrome (performed mainly for women older than 35 years).

Another method of obtaining cells from a fetus to test for CF can be done even earlier in pregnancy. This method is called chorionic villus sampling (CVS). In this procedure, a small tube is inserted through the vagina and cervix into the mother's uterus. Once the tube is in the uterus, suction is applied, and a small sample of cells from around the fetus is taken for analysis. Many families have decided to use these new methods to decide whether to continue a pregnancy or whether to stop the pregnancy (with an abortion) if the tests show that the fetus has CF. For people who would not consider having an abortion, these tests are not useful.

So far, these tests are not useful for anyone other than a couple with a CF child. DNA from blood samples from the child with CF and from each parent must be analyzed several weeks before the amniocentesis or CVS to determine whether the fetus is affected. Once the gene itself is identified, it will be possible to determine from an amniocentesis or CVS if *any* fetus has CF. For instance, if the cousin of a patient with CF wants to get pregnant, the prenatal tests currently available may not be able to tell if her baby would have CF. She and her husband would have to think about their family plans based on the statistics in the tables. In the very near future, however, a test will be available to determine if either spouse is a carrier. If it appears that both are carriers, then testing could be done to see if their baby would be born with CF. Of course, if carrier testing shows that one spouse is *not* a carrier, then no further testing would be required since both parents must be carriers for a child to be born with CF.

9 // The Family

Jean Homrighausen Zander

As a chronic disease that requires a vigorous schedule of daily treatments, cystic fibrosis (CF) imposes significant stress on the affected child, the parents, and any unaffected brothers and sisters. Understanding the reactions to this stress and learning about effective methods to cope with them are important to the care of the child with CF and to the functioning of the family.

This chapter discusses the variety of reactions to the diagnosis and management of CF, the methods for dealing with the daily stresses, and suggestions for how the family and the medical team can work together most effectively.

YOUR CHILD HAS CYSTIC FIBROSIS

Parents and other family members experience a variety of emotions when told a child has CF. Family members may say to themselves, "I can't believe this. This can't be happening to *my* child and *my* family. I don't know what to do. What does the future hold? Is there anything I can do for my child? Could I have prevented this?" All of these reactions—anger, denial, shock, grief, helplessness, confusion, despair, sadness, and fear—are very normal responses. These emotions are part of a *grieving* response. Just as a person experiences many of these feelings when a loved one dies, parents feel many of the same emotions when they learn that a child has a serious health problem. The parents "mourn" the loss of the perfect, healthy child that they had expected. Another very common response upon learning the diagnosis of CF is one of relief—if a family has taken their child to many doctors over a long period of time, they may be *relieved* finally to have been given a reason for their child's health problems. This sensation of relief may be very puzzling and the parent may even feel guilty about it.

No matter what the reaction, it's important that each family member has someone to confide in—a trusted, understanding friend or health profes-

121

sional with whom he or she can share feelings. It may be difficult for the parents to talk about CF with one another, especially immediately after the diagnosis is made. Strong emotions may make it too hard to listen and understand another person's pain, grief, or anger—even if it is a spouse. A husband and wife may find that they react very differently to the diagnosis ("how could he feel *that* way?"), making discussion even more difficult. Since they are two separate people, they may experience varying reactions at different times. This can put a strain on the relationship unless they try to remember that it is normal and that the spouse's reaction does not reflect a lack of caring. A third person may be able to help them get through this difficult time.

At the time of diagnosis, the family will be given extensive information about CF and its management. The flood of emotions may make it hard to concentrate on what the doctor is saying and to remember this information. Despite an initial lengthy discussion with the doctor, it is not uncommon for parents to retain very little of what they have been told; they may feel that they have a poor understanding of CF and have many unanswered questions.

The team at the CF center is aware that it is difficult to comprehend all this information at such a stressful time. They know that it is important to review the information many times and they plan to spend ample time with the family for this purpose.

Many parents find it helpful to write down their questions and discuss them with the doctor, nurse, or social worker during a daily conversation, in person or by phone. Typical questions that many parents ask are the following:

• Will CF affect my child's brain function?
• Will my child look any different from other children?
• How will CF affect my child's daily life?
• How long will my child live?
• Is there something I did during the pregnancy to cause my child to have CF?
• Could I have prevented this?
• Should I limit my child's activity?
• Can my child go to school?
• Do my other children have CF?

Some families are reluctant to ask these questions out of fear that they may appear insignificant or too simple. Your physician and the team members at the CF center understand and encourage the families to ask *all* their questions—no question is too insignificant to be considered.

Because manifestations of CF are so different in each child, it is often difficult for the doctor to be specific in answering many of the parents' questions. No one can predict the exact effect of cystic fibrosis on a child's lung function, growth, activity, or life span. The uncertainty is very frustrating and frightening, for it means that the family must live with the unknown from day to day. Even though the doctor cannot make any predictions for a specific child, he or she can explain to the parents the range of disease in CF and perhaps where the child falls in this range. On the whole, most children with CF should be expected to attend school regularly, to be able to participate in sports, and to play with other children without restriction.

BEGINNING HOME CARE

In addition to obtaining *information* about CF, it is important the parents learn *techniques* in caring for their child with CF—particularly the methods for respiratory treatments and enzyme administration. Many physicians recommend that the newly diagnosed infant or child be admitted to the hospital for thorough evaluation of respiratory function and growth and for education of the parents. While this idea may be frightening to the family, it often helps if they realize that an admission to the hospital provides the valuable opportunity for the parents to have daily contact with the CF team. The doctors, nurses, social worker, respiratory therapists, and dieticians use this time to teach the family about home management of CF and begin to develop an important working relationship with the family.

No matter how thorough the instructions and how skillful the parents, most families find themselves nervous about beginning therapy at home. At the same time they are beginning enzyme administration and respiratory treatments, they may be facing an already busy child-care schedule, work schedule, or both. With the help of a nurse or social worker, the parents may find it helpful to sketch out a daily schedule, which takes into consideration *their* family's needs. The doctor, nurse, or social worker may be able to arrange for a meeting with a family more experienced with CF who can serve as an important source of information and support.

In addition to the confusion of a new schedule and nervousness about new treatments, parents may find themselves faced with a cranky baby who is hard to comfort. Some babies with CF are fussy eaters, and prior to diagnosis have been irritable because of lung infection, hunger or chronic abdominal discomfort, and diarrhea. Because they have been hard to feed, hard to soothe, and haven't grown well, their parents may feel helpless and incapable.

Many parents say that they find it difficult to "like" their infant because he or she is so irritable and is frustrating to care for—and they feel guilty about resenting their own child. It may be hard for the parents to talk about these feelings or even for parents to admit them to themselves. These feelings, while very troublesome to the mother and father, are normal reactions.

Gradually, as babies become accustomed to their new medications and treatments, the chronic digestive symptoms will be relieved and they will begin to gain weight. As babies become more contented, their parents can draw much satisfaction from their daily efforts and the successful "settling in" at home.

EXPLAINING CYSTIC FIBROSIS TO OTHERS

Once they are at home, the parents must begin to explain CF to grandparents and other family members and to friends. This may be difficult to do. However, an honest, simple explanation is essential—it will set the tone for how others react to their child for many years to come. Although CF is a chronic progressive disease which may result in shortened life span, many patients live to middle age. As the prognosis for CF improves, it is important that children and teenagers be raised with the idea that they should look forward to being active, productive adults. In order to promote independence and goals for the child with CF, the parents and others with whom the child lives and works must share an outlook of hope and encouragement for the child. Many questions are difficult to answer, but each successful encounter makes the next one easier to handle.

Following are some of the important points that parents may want to share with others:

- CF does not affect the brain or intelligence.
- No part of CF, including the cough and loose stools, is contagious.
- CF is a genetic disease caused by inheriting a gene from *each* parent; it could not have been prevented and it is no one's "fault."
- CF is not curable, but it is treatable.
- The treatment for CF must be carried out each day and consists primarily of respiratory care and enzyme administration.

YOU AND YOUR SPOUSE

In conjunction with the treatment of CF, parents find themselves faced with new stresses on their marriage: care of the child takes up more time—how should they divide the responsibilities? Medicines and doctor visits are expensive—how can their budget accommodate this? There is a risk of subsequent children having CF—how can they work out their sexual relationship and family planning? The child with CF needs discipline as any other child—how should they handle discipline for a "sick" child? The other children need attention or one parent's job may be in jeopardy—how can they cope with preexisting family problems in the midst of this new stress?

An important starting point for handling each of these stresses is for the couple to be open and honest in sharing their feelings with one another. Good communication will help to define the problems from each partner's perspective, starting them on the path to developing mutually acceptable solutions. As the husband and wife work *together* to resolve conflict, many couples report that their relationship is strengthened and they are better prepared to face future challenges together.

If one spouse is employed outside the home and the other is responsible for child care, the employed spouse will probably have a limited amount of time to administer treatment. However, it is important that parents share responsibility for the child's care, even if it can only be to a limited extent. This shared responsibility demonstrates to children that their parents are unified in their approach to their care; it also may help to avoid resentment that can arise when one spouse is solely responsible for treatments.

Financial worries can cause much strain within a family. Insurance coverage may be inadequate or nonexistent. State-aid programs may be helpful in some situations. Many clinics have a "patient representative" or a social worker who can put parents in contact with appropriate financial resources.

As the husband and wife cope differently with their reactions to the diagnosis of CF, their desire for sexual intimacy may be altered. These differing needs may serve to create further conflict and misunderstanding. Overshadowing these differences may be fear of another pregnancy and the birth of another child with CF. An atmosphere of open, honest communication is essential for the resolution of these differences.

Many times the stresses associated with a diagnosis of CF are too much for a couple to handle without outside help and guidance. The Cystic Fibrosis Center team can be a valuable resource in assisting the family; they may recommend further assistance from a psychologist, counselor, or clergy. The family's pediatrician or family doctor may also be of great assistance. Although these professionals are not CF experts, they may have known the family for a long time and often are very willing to provide support. It is essential that a family seek help promptly if difficulties arise in coping with the diagnosis of CF or with related issues. Such problems do not "just go away" and must be handled directly and aggressively. Unless properly managed, problems with stress and communication within the family may persist, having an impact on CF management and adversely affecting the child's health.

GOING TO THE HOSPITAL

Occasionally, hospitalization may be necessary. Admission to the hospital upsets the daily routine of a family, and, in effect, creates a crisis. The family members must draw on new resources to cope with this stress; healthy coping patterns help the child and family to *learn* something from the experience and come away from it as stronger, more mature individuals. However, in order to accomplish this, the family must be able to rely on new resources and must be well-informed about what to expect.

Following are some questions that parents should ask in order to know what to expect in the hospital:

• What are the visiting hours?
• May I stay overnight with my child?
• May brothers and sisters visit?
• Is a "leave of absence" allowed?
• Can I assist with my child's care (baths, feeding, treatments) if I would like to do so?
• What doctor is in charge of my child's care? What other doctors will be working with him or her?
• Who are the other members of the health care team?

The child who is old enough to understand should be prepared for the hospital with simple, honest information. Questions he or she will want answered are as follows:

• How long will I be in the hospital?
• When will I go? When will I come home?
• Will I get any needle "sticks"?
• What will the other kids be like?
• Can mom and dad stay with me?

Some children may not ask questions about the hospital of their parents. They may choose to discuss their worries with another trusted adult in an effort to spare their parents additional concern. Developing relationships outside the family circle is a normal part of growing up and this should be fostered as it occurs.

Encourage the child to pack personal items from home (toys, blanket, clothes, pajamas, school books, cassette tapes and tape player) and perhaps pictures of family members. In most cases, the children should dress in their regular clothes, and should be out of bed most of the day.

The nursing staff will gather some information about the child's individual needs in order to plan his or her care. Some items that they will ask about include the child's nickname, food preferences, general likes and dislikes, favorite activities, sleeping habits, toilet habits, specific fears, and where parents can be reached.

Teaching hospitals, in which many Cystic Fibrosis Centers are located, have the advantage of providing highly skilled care by a group of specialized professionals. However, families may find the system frustrating because of the many staff members involved in their child's care. They find themselves repeating their child's medical history several times for medical students, interns, and residents. These physicians-in-training often have limited experience with CF and the parents can become upset at their lack of knowledge. Young staff members may feel threatened when faced with a knowledgeable, articulate parent and find it difficult to care for the child. Although some aspects can be trying, this is a superb opportunity: the more exposure young nurses and physicians-in-training have to CF, the more knowledgeable they will become. Since they soon will be the doctors and nurses in the community it is essential that they be as aware of CF as possible.

Parents play an important part in their child's health care and contribute their intimate knowledge of their child. Health care providers have experience with many different children over a span of years. Together, in a cooperative, positive attitude, parents and health care providers can educate one another about the needs of *this* child and effectively plan and carry out hospital care.

Most children's hospitals, and many general hospitals encourage parents to participate in their child's care but to take care to remain *parents*, not *nurses*, or *doctors* in the eyes of their child. Bathing, feeding, play and bed time stories, and maintaining normal discipline standards are activities that promote normalcy in the hospital. While parents may want to be present as a source of support and consultation during painful or frightening procedures, they should avoid being enlisted to assist directly with such procedures (such as stabilizing an arm for blood test or injection). When the latter occurs, the child may begin to associate the parent with those he sees as harming him or her and feel defenseless.

Hospitalized children have different needs of the parents at different ages. The infant and toddler are too young to understand what is occurring and cannot fully comprehend the parents' explanation. For an infant, the parents' trusted, nurturing presence can be comforting. Cuddling, rocking and singing, and playing are all familiar activities that bring security to a new, frightening environment.

As children advance to the toddler and preschool years they begin to understand more of what is occurring. Their primary fears in the hospital are abandonment and lack of mobility. They benefit from regular contact with parents and the presence of a stable group of caretakers when their parents cannot be there. They also enjoy active play, despite their IV lines!

Children in this age group have many fantasies and develop their own reasons for why things happen. They may interpret hospitalization as a punishment. New signs, smells, and sounds may be particularly frightening. They benefit from simple, concrete explanations immediately prior to the procedure about what they will *sense* (see, hear, feel, smell) during a new experience. They may also attempt to stall a nurse or doctor who is about to perform a painful procedure: as a general rule it is best to provide a simple explanation and then allow the staff member to proceed quickly and with confidence.

Preschool and school-age children have an even greater understanding of events and benefit from explanations. They also benefit from participating in planning their daily care and being provided with choices about their schedules, meals, and therapy where applicable. They should be encouraged to maintain contacts with friends while in the hospital and to develop new friendships with other patients.

Teenagers with CF are faced with the complications of a chronic illness at a time when they are most concerned with a changing body, achieving independence from the family, and establishing relationships with the opposite sex. Cystic fibrosis may thwart many of these goals by slowing growth and the development of secondary sex characteristics and by imposing a home-care regimen that perpetuates dependence on the parents. In addition, no teenager wants to "be different" from others, and the young man or woman with CF may appear different or have different needs, making it more difficult to establish new relationships. In the hospital, teenagers benefit from many of the same practices as their younger counterparts: explanations of what to expect, opportunity to participate in planning their care, making choices about some flexible areas of care, and contact with school friends. This assistance should be provided in the context of the special needs of the changing, developing adolescent who is seeking to establish some measure of independence.

When leaving the hospital it is important to get written instructions about home care and whom to call with questions and when to return for a check up.

Parents may notice some temporary changes in their child's behavior after hospitalization. Children may have nightmares, fear of strangers, fear of the parent's absence, become aggressive or rebellious, have tantrums, or try to avoid returning to school. These reactions are not unexpected but should be brought to the attention of the pediatrician or Cystic Fibrosis center team for recommendations.

10 / Cystic Fibrosis and Adulthood

David M. Orenstein

Until fairly recently, adults didn't have cystic fibrosis (CF); children had it, and they died. Today, most patients with CF live well into their adult lives. Upon reaching adulthood, people with CF must contend with some special issues, in addition to those faced by all people as they approach adulthood. Since the lung problems with CF are progressive, even though that progression can be slowed dramatically in most patients, many adults with CF will have more symptoms and limitations than they had as children and adolescents.

Patients' attitudes and outlook on life have a tremendous influence on what they are able to do, and indeed on how long they live. Patients with CF by and large have a strong, positive outlook, and therefore are able to accomplish many of the normal tasks and enjoy many of the normal pleasures of adulthood, despite having to contend with some difficulties.

MEDICAL CARE

The training of physicians in the care of adult patients with CF is just now catching up with the tremendous improvement in longevity. Until very recently, CF was a disease of childhood, and physicians who were trained to care for adults were not taught about CF. Today, there are still few internal medicine physicians (general medical specialists for adults) who have had extensive training in the problems and care of people with CF. The same is true of adult pulmonologists. Fortunately, however, there are quite a few individual physicians who have taken it upon themselves to become knowledgeable in the care of adults with CF, and medical training programs are beginning to pay more attention to the treatment of this important population. At present, the adult with CF generally has to rely on conscientious adult general medicine or pulmonary specialists who have taken the extra effort to educate themselves about CF (if it's possible to find one in your area), or continue to rely on the pediatricians and pediatric pulmonary phy-

129

sicians who have been the CF specialists for the longest time. Most CF centers have a program for their adult patients, and have physicians who are interested and knowledgeable in the care of adults with CF; in some centers these will be the pediatricians, and in others it will be internal medicine or adult pulmonary specialists.

HEALTH INSURANCE

Health insurance is a very important issue, since medical care for any chronic illness, including CF, is so expensive. Once a person reaches adulthood, he or she is usually excluded from his or her parents' family insurance coverage. Some states have "over 21" laws, which extend health insurance and/or state programs to adults with certain chronic illness, including CF. Some employers have excellent employee health insurance, but some plans exclude anyone with a "preexisting condition," meaning that they don't pay any expenses related to a problem that you had before you joined the company, which of course would include CF. Some policies have a limit to how much they pay for a particular illness; many have a lifetime limit to how much they will pay. You should find out if a hospitalization for CF at one time will count as the same "illness" as a previous hospitalization which was also due to CF. It is very important to look very carefully at insurance plans and possible exclusions before making decisions about employment.

EDUCATION

Many adults with CF choose to continue their education beyond high school, and some attend trade schools, while many graduate from college and even get advanced degrees.

One of the main ways in which CF affects an adult's education is in the decision of whether to leave home to attend college. Leaving home most often means leaving behind the people who perform daily chest physical therapy treatments, which, in turn, means that a replacement must be found. Much of the chest physical therapy can be done oneself, especially if mechanical percussors with straps or extension handles are used, but many young adults feel more secure with a treatment performed by someone else. Many college health services will offer help in this realm. Some schools which have physical therapy students or respiratory therapy students may be able to arrange for these students to help give treatments. College students often have close friends who learn how to administer treatments. Others have placed more emphasis on an aerobic exercise program or on "huff" techniques that are easier to perform on oneself than the traditional chest physical therapy. Whatever one chooses, it is extremely important to find some way to keep up with treatments, and not give in to the temptation to skip them in the excitement of being away on one's own, perhaps for the first time. There are always reasons to skip a treatment (test tomorrow, party tonight, etc.), and while it's fine to skip an occasional treatment, this cannot become a habit.

Many states have vocational rehabilitation bureaus (BVR's) which provide educational and occupational counselling and financial assistance for students after high school. These programs can be very helpful, and can help to pay for college or trade school.

EMPLOYMENT

Cystic fibrosis may well influence one's career choices. It is important to consider your current physical condition and what your physical condition will be in several years as you make occupational plans. In general, a relatively sedentary job is better than one that is physically demanding. This does not mean that a sedentary *life* is preferable, but rather that one should exercise during nonwork time. If you should become ill or weakened, then, it would not jeopardize your job and would only affect your exercise regimen. Jobs involving constant exposure to dust, chemical fumes, or smoke should be avoided.

MARRIAGE AND FAMILY

Most CF patients over 25 years of age marry, and most of these marriages succeed with a much lower divorce rate than in the general population. Decisions about raising a family are definitely difficult if one partner has a life-shortening disease that limits fertility. Women with CF have a more difficult time conceiving than women without CF, and 98 percent of men with CF are sterile. Careful consideration must be given to the potential parents' long-term health, and difficult issues must be faced such as the possible death of one parent, which would leave the other a single parent and the child or children with only one parent. If it is the woman who has CF, the possible effects of pregnancy on her health must be considered. Pregnancy has often caused dramatic deterioration in the health of women with CF if their lungs were not in excellent shape at the outset.

Quite a few women with CF have become pregnant and have had babies. Many couples in which the husband has CF have decided to adopt children, or even to have children through artificial insemination.

For the woman with CF whose lungs are not in perfect condition, avoiding pregnancy is likely to be very important for maintaining her health. Therefore, effective birth control is extremely important. Discuss the advantages and disadvantages of the various methods with your physician. The pill is the most effective method, but carries with it some risks. So-called "barrier" methods (condoms and diaphragms) are very safe, and somewhat less effective, although condoms carry with them the added advantage that they protect against transmission of some of the sexually transmitted diseases, including AIDS.

11 // Death and CF

David M. Orenstein and Denise R. Rodgers

It has been stressed throughout this book how well people live with cystic fibrosis (CF) and how much better and longer their lives are now than they were just a few decades ago. Advances in treatment and the exciting research progress promise even better things to come. In the meantime, people do still die from CF. In fact, until a cure is found, it is probable that most people with CF will die from their disease, and not of old age. In order to dispel some common misunderstandings and fears about dying, this chapter will discuss what happens when someone dies from CF.

Most people who die from CF die because their lungs have become so damaged that they can no longer perform the work of bringing in oxygen and eliminating carbon dioxide. At this point, the level of these gases in the bloodstream will be inappropriate. All body tissues need oxygen to stay alive, so when the oxygen level is too low, life is impossible. When the carbon dioxide level rises, it acts first like a sedative and then like a general anesthetic, putting the person to sleep. If the carbon dioxide levels become extremely high, the person may sleep so deeply that the breathing efforts become very weak. This can happen to such a degree that the carbon dioxide builds up even further and the oxygen drops down even further, causing the person to die.

When someone's lungs are seriously damaged, both oxygen and carbon dioxide levels may be inappropriate; however, often one of these dominates. In some people, the low oxygen level is the factor that is most apparent in their final hours or days. When this is the case, unless something is done to alter the situation, it is an extremely uncomfortable condition. "Air hunger" is a term that is used to describe how someone feels if the oxygen level is too low. This condition is very distressing, both for the patient and for family and friends who find themselves unable to relieve the suffering. Fortunately, even when the lungs are so damaged that nothing can be done to prevent the person's death, most often something *can* be done to relieve that terrible feeling.

The other problem that can occur is that the carbon dioxide level can become dangerously elevated. In this case, the high carbon dioxide level serves as a sedative, and the patient is relaxed, often asleep for much of the time. These people are not suffering. As the condition progresses, the person may fall very deeply asleep, as though under a general anesthetic. In this situation, the person may be difficult or impossible to awaken, may not respond to people in the room, and may die in his or her sleep. This is more difficult for people who are watching and waiting with the patients than for the patients themselves, since they are not uncomfortable.

WHAT CAN BE DONE?

If someone's oxygen level is low enough to be causing terrible air hunger and distress, one relatively simple thing is to give more oxygen to breathe. Although this is an obvious thing to do, it is not always done, because of physicians' concerns about its effects on how the brain controls breathing. You'll recall from Chapter 1 that when someone's lungs are badly damaged, and the carbon dioxide level has been high for some time, a low oxygen level may become the brain's main signal to keep breathing. Conscientious physicians will be concerned that if extra oxygen is given, it may raise the blood oxygen level enough that the brain will respond by inhibiting the signal to breathe hard. Breathing will then get progressively shallower, and the carbon dioxide level will build higher, putting the patient to sleep, perhaps so deeply that he or she will die.

There are several fallacies in these concerns. The first is that even when someone's carbon dioxide level has been high for some time, receiving extra oxygen *rarely* lowers the breathing level. Sometimes it even improves it (probably just by giving needed oxygen to the breathing muscles). The second essential point is that at this time, the primary concern should be for the patient's *comfort,* and sedating the person slightly by allowing the carbon dioxide to build up may, in fact, be helpful. The extra oxygen may change the situation from one in which low oxygen dominates, making the patient suffer, to one in which high carbon dioxide dominates, making the patient sedated and comfortable.

Another treatment for people who are suffering from low oxygen levels is the careful administration of a medication that can relieve the anxiety and discomfort. Morphine is the best drug for this purpose and is extremely effective. Its main danger is that too much of it can oversedate people to the point where they fall so deeply asleep that they don't wake up. Given carefully, the drug is not likely to cause this problem, and is very likely to relieve otherwise unbearable suffering. Its effects are often like those just discussed of administering oxygen: morphine and/or oxygen can sedate someone whose oxygen levels are intolerably low, making that person much more comfortable. Each medication alone or in combination with the other may also oversedate. Almost always, if a person is likely to be dying, the primary concern should be for the person's comfort.

MYTHS ABOUT DYING WITH CYSTIC FIBROSIS

There are a number of widespread misunderstandings about dying with CF which are important to mention and correct.

Choking

"My child (or I) may choke on thick mucus and die." It is certainly true that thick mucus is a problem for people with CF, and that some children and adults with CF have very hard coughing spells, where it can look (and feel) as though they won't be able to catch their breath. However, *people with CF do not die by choking on their mucus*. In fact, a sudden unexpected death in CF is extremely rare. People with CF do not go to bed well and die during the night.

Predictions

"Doctors know when a person with CF is going to die." It *is* possible to know that someone is getting sicker and that his or her pulmonary function has been declining for several months. In extreme conditions, it is even reasonable to say that someone is so sick that they are not likely to live many more hours or days. *It is never possible to be definite about the timing of death.* Physicians who have worked with CF patients for any length of time have seen patients whom they thought could not possibly make it through the night, pull through and recover sufficiently to live for months or even years longer. For this reason, many CF physicians believe that when someone is extremely ill and is unlikely to recover, it is still worth giving as much treatment as possible to enable the lungs to recover (usually IV antibiotics, aerosols, and postural drainage)—*if these treatments do not interfere with the patient's comfort.* Certainly, very invasive and uncomfortable procedures and treatments, such as using a tube in the trachea and a mechanical ventilator, are not justifiable if the chances of recovery are extremely small. On the other hand, relatively simple treatments such as IV medications, which might give a person the slight chance of recovery and which would not interfere with comfort, should be given.

Pain

"Dying from CF is very painful." If someone is dying with a very low oxygen level, that sensation of suffocation can be terrible. That sensation

can most often be lessened considerably, though, by giving oxygen, and sometimes a sedative, perhaps morphine. There is usually no physical pain.

"It's better to die at home than in the hospital."

The idea is appealing of dying among loved ones, in a familiar setting, without strangers being present and suffering intrusive treatments. This can be arranged in most hospitals, though. When the patients, family, and physician have discussed all these matters and agreed on the approach, the procedures and medications necessary to keep the patient comfortable can be handled much more readily in the hospital. For extreme circumstances, the support of the hospital staff can be very comforting to patients and their families.

"Fighting"

"It's important to keep fighting." Very often, when someone with CF is dying, that person has lived for many years (usually decades) with the disease, has done much to stay well (exercise, postural drainage treatments, medications, etc.), and has been recognized as fighting against the odds. Family, friends, and the patients themselves think of them as "fighters," in the very positive sense of that word. Too often, however, in a family's grief over losing a very special person, they may convey to that person the idea that they *must* keep fighting, and not give in. It is usually not intended this way, but the message may come across that if the patient dies, he or she has let down the family. Sometimes, after a long fight, patients may need permission to let go, and rest. They need to know that they don't have the burden of supporting their surviving family.

PATIENTS' CONCERNS ABOUT DYING

Adolescents and adults with CF (and occasionally younger children with CF) may worry about death. It is important for them to have someone to be able to talk with about these concerns. Very often they may be worried because a friend or acquaintance has died, and it may be reassuring for them to hear of ways in which they are different from the person who died, and that they are not in danger of dying soon. On the other hand, it may be that their concerns are very realistic, and that they are in fact close to the end of their lives. In either case, it is extremely important for them to be able to confide in someone, and express their fears, and have their questions answered.

It is tempting for people who care a lot about patients to reassure them, and to try to cheer them up and turn their thoughts away from death and dying. It's fine to look on the bright side of things as much as possible, but you don't do a child (or adult) a service by refusing to talk about worries on his or her mind. It may be that just listening and being supportive can relieve someone tremendously. Many people have thoughts and worries about their own death, and it is helpful for those thoughts to be openly discussed. *It is not helpful, however, to force a discussion of death on someone who is not ready for it.* Parents, close friends, physicians, and other personnel at the CF center may be the people chosen to share in this kind of discussion.

The questions that children have about death may range from whether they will be in pain (on this point they can be reassured) to whether they will see their dead relatives. A family's religious beliefs will have a strong influence on what they will want to tell children about those questions.

REACTIONS TO THE DEATH OF SOMEONE WITH CF

When a loved one dies, family and friends have many different kinds of feelings. Sadness and grief for the lost loved one, and for the suffering that he or she might have gone through, are often accompanied by feeling sorry for oneself for having to go on without the person who has died. There is also commonly a feeling of relief, especially if the death comes after a prolonged difficult period. Relief may cause guilt, but it is a perfectly normal and healthy feeling. Parents who have lost a child with CF may have some renewed sense of guilt for having "caused" the CF, or for not having done more for their child. Again, these feelings are normal, but must be balanced by the realization that *no one causes a genetic disease,* and that, in most cases, families have done an outstanding job in caring for their children. It may be time to remember that until recently, all children with CF died before school age, and if their child lived a good life beyond that, it represents an improvement, due in great part to the parents' treatment.

Parents with other children with CF may be especially sad to think that what one child has just gone through will be repeated for the surviving sibling(s). This may be true. It is also true that treatment continues to improve, and surviving children may be able to be spared some of what their sibling has just gone through.

Surviving brothers and sisters have complex reactions, which may be confusing to them. They will be sad, of course. They may have a frightening feeling that they were somehow to blame for their brother's or sister's death because of "bad thoughts" they had had. It is important for them to know that all children at some times wish that their siblings were dead, or out of the way, so that they can have their parents' attention and love. They might be feeling especially guilty because they had wished these things and had felt that their parents favored the sick child. They need to know that these thoughts are normal, and that they are not bad for thinking them, and that they did not cause their sibling's death. It can be helpful to point out ways in which the surviving child was special to the sibling who has died.

If the surviving sibling has CF, he or she may be especially frightened about his or her own fate. In this case it is helpful to point out any differences that could indicate a better prognosis for the surviving child, and to assure him or her that you and the physicians will do everything they can to keep him or her well for as long as possible. It is important not to deny the child the chance to express worries, however, and give reassurances that you'll be with him or her.

POSTMORTEM EXAMS (AUTOPSIES)

A physician may request permission for performing an autopsy. This is very difficult to think about. The postmortem exam is very important when it was not clear why the patient died. In these cases, important information may be discovered, which may make it somewhat easier for surviving family members and friends. It is also possible that something might be discovered that could benefit other children or adults with CF.

ORGAN DONATION

When someone has died, it can provide a small bit of comfort to know that he or she may still be able to help someone who is alive but suffering. Organ donations for transplantation may offer this solace. Cystic fibrosis patients have been able to donate their eyes to enable others to see, and their hearts to enable others with terminal heart disease to live.

RESEARCH

As everyone who is reading this book now knows, the basic defect for CF is not fully understood, nor is there a cure for CF, but many scientists around the world are working toward these ends. In some cases, the research can only be carried out with tissues from someone with CF. This means that it may be possible for organs from someone with CF to be donated to a research laboratory, in order to help answer the questions about CF to help future generations of people with CF.

12 / Research

David M. Orenstein

Despite the tremendous improvement in the quality and length of life of patients with cystic fibrosis (CF), there is still a long way to go in understanding the disease and in improving the treatment for it. The only way treatment will improve is through research, just as the current achievements in treatment were derived from previous research. Research into the various aspects of CF is gaining momentum lately, with some of the most creative scientists being attracted from other fields and now directing their attention to solving the many problems of CF. This chapter reviews the main areas of current research interest and progress and the direction for future research.

Research is divided into two categories—clinical and basic. Clinical research deals directly with people, examining the effects of diseases or treatments on individual patients or groups of patients. Basic research, sometimes called "bench research," concerns itself with matters that deal with tissues, cells, and even molecules, and not the whole person. Basic research provides the foundation for clinical research. Both are essential for a complete understanding and satisfactory treatment of any disease, including CF.

BASIC RESEARCH IN CYSTIC FIBROSIS

Genetics

Since CF is a genetically determined disease, finding the gene that is responsible for CF will be an important step toward unravelling the mysteries of the disease, and therefore getting closer to solving them. A new science, molecular genetics, has enabled scientists to take apart human chromosomes in the laboratory, and discover what individual tiny portions of the genetic material do. With these techniques, scientists have been able to work their way along chromosome number 7 and focus in on the section that contains the gene for CF. At the time of the publication of this book, the precise location of the CF gene has not been defined, but in all likelihood, it will be in the very near future. Once the gene has been located precisely, scientists will then be able to isolate that tiny portion of the genetic material, and work with it to determine the chemical events it directs. Once this is understood, the next step will be to find a way to undo those events without interfering with other body chemical events.

Two or three years ago, no one knew which of the 23 chromosomes contained the CF gene, and no genetic testing (for carriers or prenatal testing) was possible. Now—even before the gene itself is isolated—it is known that the gene is on chromosome 7, and many of its closer neighbors have been identified. These facts are so well established that it is possible to use these nearby genes ("markers") to tell if the family members of someone with CF are carriers, and to tell early in pregnancy whether a fetus will have CF.

Chloride Transport

Researchers in North Carolina and California recently discovered an interesting fact which may prove to be *the* defect underlying all of the problems in CF. In measuring the electrical charge inside the noses of people with CF, and then in their tracheas and bronchi, researchers noted that there was a large negative charge in people with CF. Soon afterward, they discovered the same large negative charge within the sweat duct. Normally, as fluids move through tubes and ducts in the body, sodium is pumped out of the fluid and out of the tube or duct. Sodium has a positive electrical charge, and there is a biological law which says that fluids should have as little charge as possible. Therefore, if a positive charge leaves, a negative charge usually follows along with it. In this case, the negative charge is carried by chloride. In CF tubes and ducts, the sodium (and the positive charge) is pumped out of the fluid normally, but for some reason, the negatively charged chloride does not follow—it is blocked from being transported through the wall of the tubes and ducts. In the few years that have passed since the initial descriptions of this abnormal chloride transport in the respiratory tract and sweat glands, the same phenomenon has been found to exist in the pancreas and intestines.

This is the first time in the history of CF research that a common problem has been found in all of the organs that are affected by CF. For decades, scientists described CF as a disease in which there was thick mucus in the respiratory and gastrointestinal tract, and a different problem in the sweat glands. It now is clear that all of the affected organs and glands have the same problem: chloride cannot pass through the layer of cells (the *epithelia*) on the inside walls of the tubes within the organs or glands.

It is likely that *the problem with chloride transport is the basic defect* in CF, and that it can explain all other problems seen in CF.

Exciting research is being conducted in North America as well as in other parts of the world, to figure out exactly *why* chloride cannot pass through these epithelial barriers, and why this defect leads to the problems that occur in the affected glands and organs.

Investigators in several CF research centers are working with CF tissues in laboratories to answer these critical questions. Progress has been phenomenally fast, and yet it could be even faster if it were not for several problems: it is difficult to obtain enough tissue to work with. Since animals do not get CF, the tissue must come from people with CF. Nasal polyps that are removed because they've blocked up the nose can be used, and organs could be used from patients who die. Very few patients or families are aware of this latter possibility, and often CF physicians hesitate to bring up this potentially painful topic to a grieving family around the time of the death of a patient.

Interaction Between Genetic and Transport Research

Currently, several of the laboratories working on finding the CF gene have given segments of DNA to researchers looking into the chloride transport defect. With genetic engineering techniques in the lab, they are able to substitute small segments of DNA into the tissues whose transport properties they are examining. If the segment is the segment that contains the CF gene, it should make otherwise normal tissue have the same block to chloride transport as CF tissue has.

Pseudomonas Biology

Since *Pseudomonas* colonizes and infects the bronchi of patients with CF, but not other people, the more that can be understood about the basic properties and genetics of the *Pseudomonas* bacteria, the more this problem can be understood. Several laboratories are working fulltime to answer these questions.

Mucus

Research has been conducted for several years to characterize the differences between CF and non-CF mucus. The main difference is likely to be related to chloride transport, but regardless of these findings, the researchers in this area will undoubtedly discover ways to alter CF mucus so that it will not block the bronchi and pancreatic ductules.

CLINICAL RESEARCH IN CYSTIC FIBROSIS

General

Scores of clinical research projects related to CF are continually being conducted. They may deal with any one of the problems seen with CF or its treatment. Some of the projects involve very few patients, while others involve national cooperative efforts among dozens of researchers and hundreds of patients. This chapter will review only a few of the more important areas of research, for an all-inclusive list is beyond the scope of this book.

Respiratory Research

Airway Infection

New antibiotics are constantly being developed. As they are developed, their effect in patients must be tested. At any one time there are dozens of clinical trials in which CF patients are given a course of treatment with a new antibiotic or a new combination of antibiotics to determine the effect on factors such as pulmonary function, the types and quantities of bacteria found in the sputum, exercise tolerance, and length of hospitalization.

Airway Inflammation

Since inflammation and swelling within the bronchioles and bronchi may be as important as the infection itself, research is now aimed at examining the effect of antiinflammatory medications on pulmonary function in patients with CF. Several collaborative studies are currently underway among several CF centers. At least one of these studies is designed to examine the positive and negative effects of steroids (see *Appendix B: Medications*) used on alternate days. Another study is examining the results of treatment with a nonsteroidal antiinflammatory drug (these drugs, including aspirin and ibuprofen, are commonly used for people with arthritis; they fight inflammation without the use of steroids).

Airway Obstruction

Periodically, someone performs a study to examine the effects of various techniques designed to clear mucus from the lungs (postural drainage, "huff" forced expiratory breathing maneuvers, exercise, etc.). Typically, these studies will have patients change the way they do their inhalation of aerosols, or how they perform postural drainage, and then measure pulmonary function or the amount of mucus which is spit out, to see if the new method improves pulmonary function or increases sputum clearance.

Gastrointestinal

A number of different areas have been or are being studied, including the best form of enzymes, or the best way to make enzymes work; gastroesophageal reflux in infants with CF; and ways to treat the esophageal varices that afflict the very few patients with liver cirrhosis.

Nutrition

This topic has attracted much research attention in recent years, with one result being the realization that low-fat diets, which used to be prescribed by some physicians, *are not helpful.* It has also been found that aggressive nutritional treatment, including the use of tube feedings (see Chapter 4), appears to be very beneficial for many patients, and that nutritional status is closely related to one's exercise ability and even to one's life-expectancy.

Exercise Tolerance

This is listed as its own category since it seems to be affected by many other factors, and seems to affect many other factors. Research into exercise has shown that exercise testing can be helpful in assessing a patient's progress before and after treatments of various kinds (hospitalization, exercise training programs, etc.). Exercise testing can also identify patients whose oxygen level may drop while they are active. Research in exercise tolerance has also led to the understanding that most patients with CF can exercise safely and receive the same benefits that their classmates and friends receive from a regular exercise program. Important research has also been done with regard to salt loss during exercise in the heat, leading to the recognition that people with CF can replace that salt perfectly well on their own without salt tablets or other forced salt replacement. Future research will be directed at determining the type of exercise that is most helpful for patients with CF, whether exercise can improve lung function or delay its deterioration; and the effect that improved nutrition has on exercise tolerance.

Psychology and Education

Research studies in several centers are examining the psychological adjustment of patients with CF and their families. Several studies have shown that CF patients and their families are remarkably well-adjusted, and others are directed at understanding these strengths so that people with other chronic illnesses might benefit. Additional research is focusing on the best way to educate children with CF about their illness.

RESEARCH ETHICS

Investigators' Responsibilities

Many medical researchers feel a responsibility to do what they can to answer questions that will ultimately lead to better health and less suffering for people. They also have the responsibility of conducting their research so that its drawbacks (expenditure of limited research dollars; pain and suffering of lab animals for basic research; expense, patients' inconvenience, discomfort, and possibility of toxic side effects for clinical research) are clearly outweighed by the potential benefits. All federally funded research is evaluated for the balance of risks and benefits by institutional review boards (sometimes called human rights committees) of the hospital or university where the research is taking place.

Patients who are asked to participate in research must be given complete and comprehensible explanations of the research, including its possible risks and benefits. In most cases, patients or legal guardians must sign a "consent form," saying that they do understand, and that they are participating voluntarily.

Patients' Responsibilities

Patients and families have responsibility first of all to themselves. People have an absolute right to refuse to participate in research, for whatever reason they might have. It is worth mentioning, though, that for a disease like CF, where there is no "animal model" (no animals have CF or even anything similar to it), and where there are relatively few patients with the disease (some 30,000–50,000 in the entire United States), it is essential that some people volunteer to help with research. If no one volunteers, the progress that is being made will come to a halt. Families who do participate in studies often feel that it is unfair for the burden of all the research studies to fall on a small group of people who participate time after time, while others never help. Patients associated with a large CF center are likely to have many research projects from which to choose, so they may easily participate in some, while skipping others.

SUMMARY

With the participation of many scientists and CF patients, clinical and basic research has helped answer many questions about CF and its treatment. The continued enthusiasm of researchers and patients will assure the eventual success of understanding CF completely, developing optimum treatments and—one day—finding a cure.

13 // The Cystic Fibrosis Foundation

Robert J. Beall and Sherry Keramidas

The mission of the Cystic Fibrosis Foundation (CFF) is to improve the length and quality of life for people with cystic fibrosis (CF) and to find the means to treat and control this disease. Established in 1955 by a small group of parents and caregivers of CF-affected children, the CFF is a voluntary health organization which today sponsors over 120 care centers and 12 specialized research centers. It supports dozens of universities and research institutions which are providing CF care, training, and education programs and are conducting CF-related research.

The Foundation accomplishes its goals through the direct support of programs and through collaboration with other voluntary health organizations, professional groups, government agencies, and private institutions.

ORGANIZATION OF THE FOUNDATION

The medical and scientific programs are the primary focus of the Foundation, and the Foundation is organized to take full advantage of the resources available to support these comprehensive programs.

Fund Raising

Because the Foundation receives no federal or state funds to support its programs, the Foundation has established comprehensive fund-raising programs, which are aided by public communication and education activities. The Foundation's fund raising is coordinated by the Foundation Office and implemented through national and local programs.

Field Services—Local CFF Chapters

At the heart of the Foundation are the more than 250,000 volunteers across the country who actively assist the Foundation in raising funds to support the medical/scientific programs. Organized in more than 50 chapters, these volunteers include CF-affected families, health professionals, community leaders, and other interested members of the public, who, with Foundation staff, are responsible for carrying out fund raising in their local communities.

A list of chapters is available from the Foundation office.

Medical/Scientific Programs

Because research progress is the primary thrust of the Foundation, a variety of scientific support mechanisms are used, including multidisciplinary research centers, individual basic and clinical research studies, research training programs, and large-scale clinical trials. The Foundation's other medical/scientific programs provide added breadth to pursuing the Foundation's mission.

CFF Research Centers

In 1981, the CFF launched a program to establish a network of research centers focused on CF. The concept of these centers grew from the recognition that solving a complex disease like CF requires many scientists from different fields of research, working together to find the needed answers. This program is the first such effort supported by a voluntary health organization and is endorsed by the federal government's National Institutes of Health (NIH).

By 1988, the number of research centers supported by the Foundation reached 12. Scientists at these centers are focusing on many different aspects of CF including identifying the CF gene, determining abnormalities in the cells affected by the disease, and uncovering the mechanisms of lung infection and lung damage. The work at these centers has led to major advances in understanding CF. These researchers' identification of abnormalities in the way certain biochemical substances move in and out of cells in CF lungs and sweat glands has led to the development of an important hypothesis about the disease. Moreover, the centers have been responsible for developing methods that will help scientists throughout the country further pursue the studies that may uncover the basic defect in CF. (See Chapter 12 for more about research.)

Individual Research Grants

The Foundation recognizes the importance of stimulating and supporting research by other scientists and institutions. The Foundation has pushed CF to the forefront of the scientific community by offering a number of avenues of research support in addition to the CFF research centers.

1. *Research grants* provide support for pilot and feasibility projects ranging from basic laboratory investigations to clinical management of the disease. These grants are intended to enable investigators to obtain preliminary data so that they can competitively apply for support from other agencies.
2. *New investigator research grants* attract young scientists to the CF field by supplying support while they are establishing their careers.
3. *Special research awards* are offered in response to special Requests for Applications (RFAs) by the Foundation. The objective of these awards is to direct research efforts toward specific areas of CF-related research.
4. *Clinical research grants* provide support for studies to improve clinical management of CF and to test various therapeutic approaches.
5. *Research scholar awards* encourage a sustained commitment to CF research by an individual already engaged in an independent, creative research career.
6. *CFF/NIH Awards* provide funding of highly meritorious CF-related research projects that have been submitted to and approved by the NIH but cannot be supported by available NIH funds. Support is provided for up to two years while investigators reapply to the NIH.

Fellowships

Training new investigators and caregivers to apply their talents to CF is a crucial priority of the Foundation. To that end, the Foundation offers a variety of awards for individuals interested in CF-related careers.

1. *Research fellowships* offer postdoctoral training in basic or clinical research. Preference is shown to recent graduates or those just beginning their investigative careers.
2. *Clinical fellowships* provide up to 2 years of specialized academic training for new physicians with specialties in pulmonary or gastrointestinal medicine.
3. *Third-year clinical fellowships* provide an additional year of research training for physicians who have committed themselves to specializing in CF care.

4. *NIH fellowships* are jointly sponsored by the NIH and CFF to offer advanced training with NIH staff interested in CF-related research areas.
5. *Student traineeships* are available to undergraduate and graduate students in the biomedical sciences as an introduction to the field of CF research.

Peer Review

To ensure that the Foundation uses its funds to support the best and most promising research, the Foundation has established mechanisms for carefully reviewing each proposed project. Research applications are carefully reviewed by scientific experts. Each application is judged on the quality of the science and its potential importance to understanding CF.

The Foundation also devotes considerable effort to monitoring scientific advances in many different areas and encouraging scientists to become involved in CF-related research. This is accomplished through special scientific meetings, interaction with professional societies, and preparation of materials for the scientific community. The Foundation's annual North American Cystic Fibrosis Conference attracts some 1,000 scientists and caregivers from around the world to discuss the latest advances in CF research and care.

The Foundation's efforts have contributed to a dramatic increase in the scientific interest in CF among leading researchers. This has been evident in the number of research studies submitted to and supported by the Foundation as well as the advances toward understanding CF.

Clinical Research

The Foundation's Clinical Research Program, established in 1983, uses two basic strategies to support treatment-oriented research. The first is the support of individual research studies, submitted through the Foundation's grants program and carried out at CFF care centers. Through this mechanism, the Foundation has supported studies on such topics as newborn screening, and the effects of exercise and nutrition on lung function.

The second part of this program involves large-scale clinical trials which are developed and managed by the Foundation and its medical advisors. The studies in this category involve the participation of many CFF care centers and a large number of individuals with CF. These trials generally represent the final stage of studying promising new treatments before their translation into standard medical care. In 1986, the Foundation initiated its first collaborative study involving 13 CFF care centers and 300 patients. Additional large-scale studies are now underway and more will be initiated.

CFF Care Centers

The CFF Care Center Program is a nationwide network of more than 120 medical institutions (see Appendix E) where individuals with CF and their families can seek diagnosis, comprehensive specialized care, and long-term follow-up from professionals knowledgeable in the latest advances in CF treatment. Most centers are associated with medical schools and teaching hospitals and offer a range of outpatient and inpatient services.

Centers that are part of this care network must meet specific requirements in terms of staff, facility, and service. Centers are regularly reviewed by a group of the Foundation's medical advisors. Staff of these care centers often have specialized training related to CF. In addition, the Foundation keeps these professionals up to date on research and advances in care through special meetings and publications.

The CFF care centers are a key source of care and support for individuals with CF and their families. In addition, these centers are an important resource for research on CF and provide the environment for conducting clinical research on new treatments. Further, the CFF care centers are an important part of the education and training of health professionals who are interested in CF.

PARTNERSHIP WITH THE NATIONAL INSTITUTES OF HEALTH

Beyond the Foundation, research related to CF is also funded by the NIH, the leading supporter of biochemical research in the world. The Foundation has carefully designed its programs to complement those CF-related programs of the NIH. In addition, the Foundation interacts regularly with the staff of the NIH to identify additional research opportunities related to CF and to encourage scientific interest in these areas. The Foundation's efforts have led to a large series of NIH research meetings on CF and to a dramatic increase in the NIH support of CF studies.

In 1988, NIH support of CF-related research was more than $25 million. The Foundation will continue to work closely with the NIH to identify research opportunities and to support promising new studies.

OTHER FOUNDATION EFFORTS TO IMPROVE QUALITY OF LIFE

The Foundation's consumer affairs and public policy programs address the social concerns and public policy issues that affect individuals with CF. The Foundation actively participates in developing and monitoring legislation at the federal and state levels to promote and protect the needs of people with CF and their families. These efforts have included encouraging legislation and funds for pooled risk health insurance programs, "Over-21" programs offering medical assistance to adults with CF, and medical reimbursement.

Representatives from the Foundation also have been invited annually to testify before congressional committees considering health care issues and budget appropriations for the NIH.

The Consumer Affairs Program also addresses the needs of adults with CF. Through direct contact with Foundation staff and through the Foundation's educational pamphlets, adults with CF can obtain information on college, employment, health care, and other concerns of this growing CF adult population. The Foundation also sponsors a summer intern program for adults with CF at various Foundation offices, to provide professional experience in a variety of fields.

DIRECTIONS FOR THE FUTURE

Recent scientific strides toward understanding the genetic and cellular abnormalities in CF have created a new momentum in the scientific community and in the Foundation. Cystic fibrosis is no longer a little-known disease; rather, research on CF is at the forefront of scientific interest. Newspapers, magazines, and television frequently carry stories about CF and the research efforts to control this disease.

Although it is impossible to predict when medical research will provide the answers needed to control CF, the Foundation is approaching the future with an increasing sense of optimism, challenge, and vigor. The Foundation will continue its emphasis on research to understand CF and to develop therapies that will improve further the life of individuals with CF. Inherent in this strategy, the Foundation will continue to stimulate new and innovative research and to involve outstanding scientists in this effort.

To support its aggressive medical/scientific plans, the Foundation is implementing new approaches to raising funds at the local and national levels. To be even more effective, the Foundation also is seeking to involve more members of the community in its chapters.

The future directions of the Foundation will continue to be shaped by its ultimate goal—to find a cure for cystic fibrosis. The outlook for individuals affected by this disease grows brighter every day. The ingredients necessary to reach the Foundation's goal—the base of scientific knowledge, the research technologies and the medical/scientific manpower—are now available. Research continues to progress as the Foundation seeks the answers needed to conquer this disease.

Glossary of Terms

aerosol A mist for inhalation, usually containing medicine. Aerosol mists may be made by an air compressor that blows air through a *nebulizer* which contains liquid medicine, or may come from a handheld spray can.

airways The tubes that carry air in and out of the lungs. These tubes begin with the nose and mouth and include the trachea (windpipe), bronchi, and bronchioles.

alveoli The air sacs of the lung where gas exchange takes place.

anorexia Loss of appetite.

atelectasis Incomplete expansion of a portion of the lung, usually caused by mucous plugging.

b.i.d. An abbreviation meaning "twice a day."

baseline One's normal state of health. The baseline or usual level of functioning includes a number of considerations, such as the amount of cough, exercise tolerance, and breathing effort. One's baseline health is often referred to for comparison. For example, after a pulmonary exacerbation, the goal of treatment is to return someone to his or her baseline state of health.

bicarbonate An acid-neutralizing juice that is normally produced by the pancreas.

blood gas The level of oxygen and carbon dioxide in the bloodstream, especially in the arteries. The term "blood gas" is also used to refer to the test and to the actual measurement of oxygen and carbon dioxide.

bronchi The tubes through which air travels between the trachea and the bronchioles.

bronchioles The smallest airways, connecting the bronchi to the alveoli. These airways differ from the bronchi in that they are smaller and have no cartilage to support them.

bronchus Singular of bronchi.

cardiovascular system The heart and blood vessels.

central line A kind of intravenous catheter that extends into a very large vein, or even into the heart.

cilia The tiny hairs in the nose, trachea, and bronchi, which, through their coordinated movement, help keep the airways clean.

clubbing An abnormal shape to the tips of the fingers and toes, which is associated with many different conditions, including cystic fibrosis.

cyst A fluid-filled sac.

diaphragm The main breathing muscle. The diaphragm is located at the bottom of the lungs, and separates the chest from the abdomen.

digestion The process of breaking foods down into particles that are small enough to be absorbed through the intestinal wall into the bloodstream.

ectasia Abnormal distention or enlargement. Bronchi*ectasis* is abnormal widening of the bronchi.

-emia A suffix meaning "in the blood." Thus, hypox*emia* means lower than normal oxygen level in the blood.

enzymes Chemicals that help perform biologic processes in the body; "enzymes" usually refer to digestive enzymes, which are the chemicals formed in the pancreas which break down food into absorbable particles.

esophagus The tube that connects the mouth to the stomach.

fellow A physician in training for a subspecialty. A fellow has completed medical school, internship, and a specialty residency.

fibrosis Scarring.

flaring Nasal flaring.

gas exchange The process of bringing oxygen into the bloodstream and removing carbon dioxide.

gastrostomy A surgical opening through the abdominal wall into the stomach. A tube is placed through this opening, which allows feedings to be given through the tube.

GE reflux Gastroesophageal reflux. A process in which fluid moves backwards from the stomach into the esophagus.

heart failure A condition in which the heart is not able to pump its full load of blood, resulting in the backup of fluid. Heart failure is *not* heart stoppage.

hemoptysis Coughing up blood.

hep lock (*see* Glossary of Drugs in Appendix B) An intravenous needle whose end can be plugged while it is not being used for medication administration.

hyper A prefix meaning "more than normal." Thus, a *hyper*active child is more active than normal.

hyperalimentation This term literally means "over-feeding," but actually refers to the method of giving extra nutrition through an IV.

hypo A prefix meaning "less than normal." Thus, *hypo*xia means less oxygen than normal.

I.M. Intramuscular. A way of administering medicine by injection into the muscle.

intern A physician who has graduated from medical school, and is training in a medical specialty such as pediatrics, internal medicine, family medicine, or surgery.

internal medicine The branch of medicine dealing with the general health of adults.

internist   A medical specialist in internal medicine (not to be confused with an *intern*).

-itis   A suffix meaning "inflammation." Thus, bronch*itis* means inflammation of the bronchi.

jejunum   The second part of the small intestine.

jejunostomy   A surgical opening made through the abdominal wall into the jejunum. This opening is used to hold a tube for feedings, as is a gastrostomy.

larynx   The part of the upper airway that contains the vocal cords—the "voicebox."

lobe   The largest division of the lung. The right lung has three lobes and the left has two.

mucociliary escalator   A mechanism for keeping the lungs clear. Particles get trapped in the mucus, and the cilia move the mucus out of the lungs.

mucous   Having properties like mucus. ("Mucus" is a noun; "mucous" is an adjective.)

mucus   The slimy fluid secreted in many glands of the body, and whose function appears to be to protect and lubricate.

nasal flaring   Widening of the nostrils with each breath (often abbreviated, "flaring"). This is a sign that someone is working harder than normal to breathe.

nebulizer   A device used with an air compressor which directs the compressed air past liquid medication, lifting the medication into a mist ("aerosol") for inhalation (*see* page 23).

NG tube   Nasogastric tube. A tube that passes through the nose into the stomach. This tube is used for feeding someone who can't eat, for continuous feeding during sleep, or for the administration of other substances such as medicines.

peak   The highest level that a drug reaches in the bloodstream.

PFT   Pulmonary function test (see Chapter 1).

pneumothorax   Collapsed lung caused by a hole in the lung. Air escapes from the lung through this hole, collects within the chest, and presses in on the lung.

pulmonary exacerbation   An episode of worsening of the lung disease, usually caused by worsened bronchial infection.

pulmonology   The branch of medicine dealing with breathing problems.

reflux   The backwards movement of fluid; this term is often used to refer to *gastroesophageal reflux*.

resident   A physician who has completed medical school and is undertaking further training in a medical specialty.

resistant   This term means "not killed by" when used to describe bacteria's relation to an antibiotic. For example, the statement, "*Pseudomonas* bacteria are resistant to penicillin," means that, in the lab, penicillin does not readily kill *Pseudomonas*.

respiratory failure   The condition in which blood oxygen levels are too low and blood carbon dioxide levels are too high.

retracting   The pulling in of skin between the ribs with each breath, indicating hard breathing.

saline   Salt water (see Appendix B).

segment   The second largest division of the lung. Each lobe is divided into several segments.

sensitive   This term means "killed by" when used to describe bacteria's relation to an antibiotic. For example, the statement, "*Strep* bacteria are sensitive to penicillin," means that, in the lab, penicillin kills *Strep*.

specialty (*or* **medical specialty**)   One of the main branches of medical practice in which physicians can become trained and qualified. The specialties are pediatrics, internal (adult) medicine, obstetrics/gynecology, surgery, psychiatry, and family medicine. Physicians may focus their skills and training in more specialized areas, called **subspecialties**, such as pediatric pulmonology, cardiology, and neurosurgery. (A pediatric pulmonary specialist must first become a pediatrician; a neurosurgeon must first become a surgeon.)

sputum   Mucus from the lungs which is coughed up and spit out.

stoma   A hole, usually one created purposely by a surgical procedure. This word is often used as a suffix: tracheo*stomy* is a hole made in the trachea; gastro*stomy* is a hole through the abdominal wall into the stomach.

toxicity   Harmful effect(s). This term is often used to refer to the undesirable effects of a medication.

TPN   Total parenteral nutrition. This term refers to nutrition given through an IV (same meaning as *hyperalimentation*).

trachea   The tube that carries air from the mouth and throat into the chest, where it connects with the bronchi from each lung.

tracheostomy   A hole placed in the trachea.

trough   The lowest level that a drug reaches in the bloodstream (this level is found immediately preceding a dose of the drug).

ventricle   One of the two main portions of the heart. The right ventricle pumps blood through the lungs, and the left ventricle then pumps the blood to the rest of the body.

B // Medications

Your physician knows the most about your treatment needs and will prescribe the best medications for you. *No medications should be taken without the advice of your physician.* Contact your physician if you have questions about the medications described.

INTRODUCTION

This appendix is organized according to the systems of the body; for example, the antibiotics used to combat lung infection are discussed under *Respiratory System Medications: Lungs,* and digestive enzymes are discussed under *Gastrointestinal and Digestive System.* For each medicine discussed, there is information on how the drug is taken as well as possible side effects or dangers.

The most common method of taking the drugs described in this appendix is by mouth. Some medicines can be given by injecting them into a vein (IV, for *In*tra*V*enous injection) or into a muscle (IM). Others can be breathed into the lungs, or sniffed into the nostril, while still others may be applied directly to the skin.

A word about side effects: Every medicine has *potentially* serious side effects. There is *no* drug that has only good effects, and absolutely no dangers. However, all the drugs discussed here have passed numerous tests, which, to most doctors and scientists, will mean that the drug's benefits outweigh their risks. Most people are able to take most of the medicines in this book without experiencing any serious problems. The "undesirable effects" noted for each drug are not meant to frighten you but to help you be as well informed as possible about your medications.

Drug names (generic names and the trade names given by the drug companies) are listed in the *Glossary of Drugs* at the end of Appendix B.

RESPIRATORY SYSTEM MEDICATIONS

Lungs

Antibiotics

Antibiotics are drugs used to fight infections caused by bacteria. They do not kill other kinds of germs, such as viruses and fungi. There are many different families of

157

antibiotics, several methods of taking antibiotics, and certain unwelcome effects with which you should be familiar. These areas are all discussed below.

Penicillins

This family was first used in the early 1940s and was one of the earliest groups of drugs to be used to fight infection in people. The number of drugs included in this family has grown tremendously over the past 30 years. New members of the penicillin family keep appearing, so it is impossible to list them all. Although the members of the penicillin family have distinct, individual personalities, there are a number of shared characteristics. The most important of these is that if you are allergic to any one penicillin, there is a strong chance that you will be allergic to all of them.

1. PENICILLIN. The first in its family (as you might have guessed from the name), this drugs kills many germs, especially *Streptococcus* (*Strep*) and *Pneumococcus* (the "pneumonia germ"). However, these bacteria are not the major problem bacteria for CF patients. The most common causes of CF patients' bronchial infections are *Hemophilus, Staphylococcus* (*Staph*), or *Pseudomonas,* and penicillin is usually not effective in treating these infections.

   How taken: Penicillin can be given by mouth, by IV, or IM.

   Undesirable effects: Allergic reactions to penicillin can be mild, but can also be very serious. Any of the drugs in this family can cause a reaction in someone who is allergic to penicillin. Penicillin injections are painful. Other than these two problems, penicillin is remarkably gentle to the human body while being brutally hard on the unwelcome bacteria.

2. AMPICILLIN. Ampicillin kills *Hemophilus* (also called *H. flu*) in addition to the bacteria which penicillin kills. It does not usually kill *Staph* or *Pseudomonas*.

   How taken: Ampicillin is most commonly taken by mouth. It can also be given by IV or IM injection.

   Undesirable effects: Loose stools are fairly common in people taking oral ampicillin. A skin rash may appear in some people, too, even if they are not actually allergic to the penicillins.

3. AMOXICILLIN. This is a slightly different version of ampicillin; it kills the same bacteria, but is only given by mouth, and is less likely to cause diarrhea.

4. AUGMENTIN. This combines amoxicillin with another chemical, clavulanic acid, and makes it effective against *Staph* in addition to the usual bacteria which are killed by amoxicillin.

5. METHICILLIN, OXACILLIN, NAFCILLIN. These three drugs have been modified so that they kill *Staph* very well. They do not usually kill *Hemophilus* or *Pseudomonas*.

   How taken: These drugs are used mostly by IV, but can also be given IM. Oxacillin and nafcillin have some effect if taken orally (but not as much as cloxacillin or dicloxacillin, discussed next).

   Undesirable effects: These drugs are irritating to the tissues where they are injected. They can cause discomfort as they go into a vein.

6. CLOXACILLIN, DICLOXACILLIN. These are also good anti-*Staph* drugs, used only by mouth. Otherwise they are similar to the other anti-*Staph* penicillins.

7. CARBENICILLIN, TICARCILLIN, PIPERACILLIN, MEZLOCILLIN, AZLOCILLIN. These are anti-*Pseudomonas* drugs. They generally do not kill *Staph,* but they do kill *Hemophilus.*

How taken: Almost always given IV. They can be given IM, but most people feel this is not a practical way to administer the drugs over the relatively long period of time (1–3 weeks or longer) for which they are usually used. Carbenicillin can also be given by mouth for treating bladder infections, but none of the drug gets to the lungs if it's taken by mouth. Therefore, orally, it is not effective in treating CF *Pseudomonas* bronchial infections. Occasionally, these drugs are given by inhalation.

Undesirable effects: In addition to the possibility of allergic reactions in people who are allergic to penicillin, and the irritation these drugs can cause when they are injected, there are some other problems which occasionally arise. These medicines can make liver tests appear abnormal; fortunately, however, the problem is only with the lab result and not with the liver itself. The liver continues to function normally, and if the medicine continues to be given, the tests will return to normal. These antibiotics can also interfere with the function of platelets (blood cells which are responsible for proper clotting of blood).

8. TIMENTIN. This combines ticarcillin with clavulanic acid, the way Augmentin combines it with amoxicillin, to make the ticarcillin effective against *Staph* in addition to *Pseudomonas* and *Hemophilus.*

Sulfa Drugs

These were the first antibiotics ever used to fight infections in people, and they still have many uses.

1. SULFISOXAZOLE. This drug can help in some infections with *Hemophilus,* but it is of no use in fighting *Pseudomonas.*

How taken: By mouth.

Undesirable effects: Problems with this drug are not common. Some people have allergic skin reactions.

2. TRIMETHOPRIM–SULFAMETHOXAZOLE (TMP–SMX). This is a combination of two drugs. Trimethoprim is not a sulfa drug, but the combination is quite effective in treating several kinds of bacteria, usually including *Hemophilus.* It is not usually effective for infections caused by *Staph* or *Pseudomonas.*

Aminoglycosides

This family includes gentamicin, tobramycin, neomycin, kanamycin, amikacin, and netilmicin. Many kinds of *Pseudomonas* infections can be treated effectively with these drugs, especially with gentamicin, tobramycin, amikacin, and netilmicin.

These drugs seem to be particularly helpful in killing *Pseudomonas* if they are given with an anti-*Pseudomonas* penicillin.

How taken: Almost always given by IV or IM injection since these antibiotics are not absorbed well into the bloodstream if they are taken by mouth. Shots into the muscle with these drugs are not as painful as with the penicillins. These drugs have also been used by inhalation.

Undesirable effects: The two main problems with these drugs are their effects on the kidney and the ears. These problems are usually (but not always) avoidable if the blood levels of the drug are checked and dosages adjusted to keep the blood levels in what is considered to be the safe range. The kidney problems are usually just abnormal lab results, and are not uncomfortable for the patient. The ear problem is worsened hearing. The harmful kidney effects almost always disappear if the drug is stopped (or the dosage reduced). If the drugs are continued after the hearing or kidney damage has begun, there can sometimes be serious and permanent damage.

Chloramphenicol

This is one of the most powerful and effective antibiotics available for use in CF patients. It kills *Hemophilus,* some *Staph,* and another family of bacteria called anaerobes (bacteria that live without oxygen). It generally does not kill *Pseudomonas*. Despite this fact, it often is helpful in CF patients whose main infection seems to be *Pseudomonas*. It is not known if this is because those patients have other bacteria which are not found on culture (like the anaerobes, which are difficult to culture in the lab). Because of its serious side effects, it should never be taken without your doctor's direct instruction.

How taken: By mouth or IV.

Undesirable effects: This drug has developed a bad reputation because of some real dangers and because of a lot of misuse. Some pharmacists who are not aware of its benefits in CF patients may even try to convince you not to take it! There are two main problems with chloramphenicol, both having to do with the body's production of blood: in rare instances (less than one case in 40,000 courses of treatment), the production of blood cells may be shut off completely and irreversibly. If this happens, it is nearly always fatal. Another much more common blood-production problem is that, in many people, taking large doses for more than 2 weeks can result in the slowing down of the production of blood cells and lead to anemia. This problem is very different from the complete shut off of blood production, for this slow production always returns to normal after the drug is stopped. Most doctors check blood counts in their patients on "chloro" to detect if blood cell production is slowing down. There are a few other less common, nuisance-type problems, including a tingling feeling in the fingers and some rashes. Rarely, it can cause blurry vision and very rarely, blindness. Most of the serious problems with chloramphenicol have arisen when it is used inappropriately. Furthermore, there is strong evidence that this drug can be extremely effective in treating patients with CF lung infection when other antibiotics have not helped. Most CF doctors feel that the strong chances of its helping to stop or limit lung damage outweigh the small chance of a serious problem with it.

Cephalosporins

This family of antibiotics is growing even faster than the penicillins. Most members of this family are helpful in combatting infections with *Strep, Staph,* and *Hemophilus.* Some of the newest members of this family have some activity against *Pseudomonas.* To preserve space, only a few of the more commonly used cephalosporins are listed here (but a more complete listing is in the glossary). Cephalexin and cefaclor are both taken by mouth only. Cephalothin, cephaloridine, ceftazidime, and ceftaxime are given only by injection (IM or IV).

Undesirable effects: About one-third of people who are allergic to penicillins will also be allergic to cephalosporins. Other problems are fortunately not common, but include diarrhea or other stomach/intestinal upset.

Erythromycin

These drugs are most commonly substituted for penicillin in people who are allergic to penicillin. They kill *Strep,* many *Staph* and *Hemophilus,* and several other bacteria which aren't big problems in CF. However, they do not fight *Pseudomonas.*

How taken: Erythromycins are most often taken by mouth, but IV forms are also available.

Undesirable effects: Abdominal cramping is sometimes an effect of these drugs, and some years ago there was a scare about liver damage with some erythromycin preparations. It now seems that liver damage is not very likely with this medicine.

Tetracyclines

The tetracyclines were among the first drugs available which had any effect against *Pseudomonas.* They are no longer as helpful as they once were because many bacteria have become resistant to their effects. There are still some *Pseudomonas, Staph, Hemophilus,* and *Strep* bacteria which are sensitive to tetracyclines.

How taken: The tetracyclines are usually taken by mouth, but can be given by IV or IM injection.

Undesirable effects: The main undesirable effect of tetracycline, one that's known to those CF patients in their 20's, is that if it's given between the ages of approximately 4 months and 8 years, it can permanently stain the teeth a grayish/brownish/yellow color. Fifteen years ago, physicians knew about the tooth problem, but often didn't have any other antibiotics to give, so they had to use a tetracycline. Fortunately, today there usually is another antibiotic available, and tetracycline should almost never be used in young children. Other side effects include allergic reactions, intestinal upset, and a rash which is made worse by being exposed to the sun.

Quinolones

This family of antibiotics has some activity against *Pseudomonas* in the lung, even when the drugs (especially ciprofloxacin) are taken by mouth.

How taken: Several of these medications can be taken by mouth.

Undesirable effects: Remarkably few side effects have been recognized with these new antibiotics. As they are used longer, some side effects may appear. To date, intestinal upset has been seen occasionally. Another problem seems to be that bacteria become resistant to the quinolones very soon after the patient starts to take them (within a week or two). Young animals given these drugs have developed some problems with the cartilage in their joints, so most physicians are reluctant to prescribe the drugs for young children.

Aztreonam

This drug is one with some anti-*Pseudomonas* activity; it is relatively new, and therefore there is not much experience with it, but it seems to be safe and effective.

How taken: Aztreonam is taken by IV injection.

Undesirable effects: The side effects of this drug have been few and not very serious. They have included diarrhea, nausea, allergic reactions, and tenderness at the site of injection.

Perhaps two final words should be said about antibiotics and undesirable effects: the first is that antibiotics kill or control bacteria; that is their job, and they are usually very good at it. However, antibiotics can't tell good bacteria from bad. Everyone does have some good bacteria in the body, especially in the mouth and intestines. Among other things, these good bacteria keep people from becoming overrun with funguses and yeasts. Sometimes while someone takes antibiotics, the good bacteria are killed along with the bad. When this happens, a yeast infection can take hold, with a cheesy-looking material in the mouth ("thrush") or vagina. Generally, these yeast infections are easily dealt with, but your doctor needs to know about them in order to prescribe the right medicine (usually nystatin). The same problem of killing the good bacteria can also cause trouble in the intestines, and some patients develop diarrhea from antibiotics.

The last point to mention is that with the availability of so many new medicines, it is possible that new side effects can appear which have not been seen or recorded. If you develop *any* disturbing symptoms or problems shortly after you've started taking a new antibiotic, it may be from the new drug and you should let your doctor know about it.

Bronchodilators ("Asthma Medicines")

Some people with CF also have asthma, or a condition like asthma, where the bronchi can become partly blocked for a time when the muscles surrounding the bronchi squeeze down. Bronchodilators are medicines that open (dilate) the bronchi by relaxing the muscles around them. The medicines are effective in treating bronchospasm once it starts and help to prevent it from occurring. Some of these drugs can be taken by inhalation, some by injection (either IM, IV, or under the skin), some by mouth, and some by several different methods. Bronchodilators seem to help some people with CF, while not being effective in others.

Theophyllines

This family of bronchodilators is a large and excellent one. However, there may be some confusion dealing with dosages and preparations, since almost every drug company has its own version of theophylline, with a similar name but different dosage. In addition, people process theophyllines at different speeds. In one person, 100 mg may reach a good level in the bloodstream and stay there for a long time, while in another, it may give only a low level and be gone quickly. For this reason, doctors often like to check a blood level of theophylline, to see if someone needs more or less than the average to reach a level in the bloodstream that is effective and safe.

Some theophyllines are short-acting, and are eliminated from the body quickly. Others are released slowly, and stay in the body longer. The short-acting theophyllines usually need to be given 4 times a day (about every 6 hours), while the slow-release or sustained-release kind can be given 3 times a day (every 8 hours), or even (especially for older children, adolescents, and adults) twice a day, and still keep a good blood level for many hours.

How given: Theophylline can be given in the vein ("aminophylline"), or by mouth as a liquid, tablet, or capsule. There are preparations that can be given rectally, like an enema. Usually the rectal kind is not as safe, since it's harder to predict just how much will be absorbed into the bloodstream.

Undesirable effects: There are two main side effects: some people get stomach upset with this family of medicines, and may lose their appetite, or even vomit. Nausea or vomiting can be important signs that the person is getting too much theophylline. People with CF may be more likely than other people to have this stomach upset with theophyllines. Some children also become agitated or overactive when they get too much of this drug. These side effects are quite common. However, if the drug is started (or restarted) at a very low dose, then raised very slowly, most people will be able to tolerate relatively high levels of the drug. A very large overdose can cause seizures (convulsions), a danger which, fortunately, is rare.

Beta-Agonists

This is the name applied to a class of very helpful bronchodilators, including Bronkosol, Metaprel, Alupent, Ventolin, and others.

How taken: These drugs can be taken by injection, by mouth (pills or liquids), or by inhalation (either from a hand-held cannister-type nebulizer, or from the air-compressor type of aerosol machine).

Undesirable effects: The three main undesirable effects of this class of drugs are: (1) jitteriness, which often goes away with continued use of the drugs; (2) overactiveness (getting "hyper"), a side effect seen much less often with these drugs than with theophylline; and (3) stimulation of the heart, causing it to speed up, which can be somewhat annoying. It may also cause an irregular heart beat, which can be dangerous. Dangerous effects are uncommon if the drugs are taken by mouth or by inhalation. In the 1960s, a number of deaths were reported in patients with asthma who used their hand-held nebulizers of beta-agonists too much. It's not clear what caused these deaths, but there are two likely reasons: it may have been the chemical used to make the aerosol, and not the bronchodilator itself; or, it may have been that patients got such good relief from the inhalations that they didn't see their doctor for a very serious asthma attack, but instead kept puffing on their aerosols, even when the effect lasted a shorter and shorter time. When they finally did try to go for help, they were too sick. Today, the vehicle for delivering the aerosol is safer. However, there is still a danger if a patient with asthma or CF tries home-prescribed antibiotics, bronchodilators, etc. While they may seem to work at first, they can lead to serious consequences. Talk to your doctors about medicine changes, in order to avoid dangerous combinations or dosages.

Cromolyn

This drug doesn't actually relax the muscles around the bronchi, but may be very effective in preventing certain bronchoconstricting chemicals from being released in the body. It seems to help about 60 percent of patients with asthma or asthma-like conditions. There is no way of telling which patients will be helped by it, except by trying.

How taken: This drug is almost always taken by inhalation, either from a powder within a capsule which is punctured inside a hand-held "spinhaler," from a liquid aerosolized in a regular air compressor/nebulizer, or from a hand-held metered-dose inhaler.

Undesirable effects: A few patients may have some bronchial irritation from this medicine if it's inhaled in the powdered form. Otherwise, it is unlikely to cause any trouble.

Steroids

Steroids, also called "corticosteroids," are cortisone-like drugs whose name strikes fear in the hearts of many people because of the serious side effects caused by improper use. Actually, steroids can be extremely useful and very safe if used properly. In fact, everyone's body makes these drugs themselves and they are extremely important in maintaining health. It is not clear exactly how they work in asthma, but they seem to increase the sensitivity of the body to the effects of the beta drugs. They also probably decrease inflammation and swelling within the bronchi.

How taken: Steroids can be taken by mouth (pills or liquid), by IV injection, or by inhalation. One kind of inhaled steroid, beclomethasone or triamcinolone, seems to affect the bronchi by preventing bronchoconstriction, not really reversing it once it's started. This form has very little toxic effect on the rest of the body. There are many different schedules for taking steroids. They can be given several times a day, once a day, or once every other day. They can be given for a brief period—a 3–5 day "burst"—or for months. The schedule depends on the drug being used, what it is being used for, and the characteristics and needs of the person taking it.

Undesirable effects: There are many possible effects including greatly increased appetite and swelling, decreased growth in height, increased possibility of developing diabetes, bone brittleness, and difficulty in fighting infection. In general, the lower the dose and the shorter the length of time steroids are given the less likely one is to develop side effects. When these drugs are used for longer than a week, the body begins to detect them and seem to say, "Well, we don't need to make any more of our own." If the drug is then stopped abruptly, the body is left without the protection of its own steroids. For this reason, if steroids are required for more than 6 or 7 days, you can't suddenly just stop the drug; instead, you need to reduce (taper) the amount you take over several days or even weeks (depending on how long you've been on them, and how used your body has become to receiving them from an outside source) so that your body gradually gets used to the idea of having to make steroids on its own again. If the drugs are used for less than a week, they can be stopped abruptly with an extremely small likelihood of side effects. Another way to get around most of the side effects is to take the drugs every other day. This gives the body a day to recover between doses. Of course, in some cases, when steroids are really needed, a patient may not be able to tolerate being off them for that in-between day.

Mucolytics

"Lysis" means destruction or decomposition of a substance, so mucolytics are drugs that destroy or break down mucus. Since much of the lung trouble in CF has to do with extra-thick mucus, a completely safe and completely effective mucolytic for the lung would be wonderful. There isn't such a drug right now. However, when one drug, acetylcysteine (Mucomyst) is put in a glass test tube with CF lung mucus, it breaks down the mucus, making it much more watery, and easier to move. It doesn't work quite that well in the body, but it does seem to help some patients.

How taken: This drug is almost always given by inhalation, and is probably not effective given any other way.

Undesirable effects: In many people this drug causes bronchial irritation with production of more mucus. In others, it causes bronchospasm. Some physicians prescribe an aerosolized bronchodilator along with Mucomyst to try to prevent bronchospasm. Mucomyst smells like rotten eggs and is expensive.

Oxygen

Most people with CF don't need any more oxygen than the amount that is in the regular air around us. Air is 21 percent oxygen, and at sea level this generally provides plenty of oxygen for most people's bodies. If the lungs are severely affected by disease, or when someone is at high altitude, or when someone with moderate lung disease is exercising, it may be difficult for enough oxygen to enter the bloodstream. In these cases, people can breathe extra oxygen—air with 25, 30, 40 percent or more oxygen. When someone's blood oxygen level is very low, it is remarkable how much better a little extra oxygen can make him or her feel.

How given: Oxygen can be kept in metal cylinders of different sizes. Small "B-cylinders" are about 3½ inches across and 16 inches high, and weigh about six pounds when full. If someone is using 5 liters/minute (see below), these cylinders last 44 minutes. Other cylinders are as follows:

Cylinder time (at 5 liters/min)	Size	Weight (full)
B: 44 min.	3½″ × 16″	6 lbs.
D: 70 min.	4¼″ × 20″	10 lbs.
E: 2 hrs.	4¼″ × 30″	14 lbs.
M: 11 hrs.	7⅛″ × 46″	82 lbs.
G: 17 hrs.	9″ × 51″	127 lbs.
K: 23 hrs.	9″ × 55″	150 lbs.

Oxygen can also be stored in liquid form. Liquid oxygen tanks hold much more oxygen in the same space than oxygen gas. Different sized tanks of liquid oxygen are also available:

Cylinder time (at 5 liters/min)	Size	Weight (full)
Stroller: 3½ hrs.	13½″ Oval	9.5 lbs.
L-30: 86 hrs.	12″ × 35″	120 lbs.

One other way of giving extra oxygen in the home is with an oxygen extractor or concentrator, which takes in regular room air and gets rid of the parts of air that are not oxygen (mostly nitrogen), resulting in almost pure oxygen. This method is expensive, and the machines are fairly bulky and somewhat noisy, but for someone who needs oxygen much of the time, it may be cheaper and more convenient than using many small tanks.

Just how much extra oxygen you breathe depends on how the oxygen gets from the tank to your lungs. The main methods are mask and nasal cannula. The mask takes the pure oxygen from the tank and mixes it with varying amounts of room air to deliver 25, 30, 35, 50, or even 100 percent oxygen. Nasal cannulas, which consist of a flexible plastic tube with two short plastic prongs at the end which stick a short way into the nostrils, can deliver different amounts depending on how high you set the flow of oxygen from the tanks: for every liter per minute of oxygen flow, you add about 3–4 percent oxygen above room air. That means that if the flow is set at 4 liters/minute, you get 4 × 3 = 12 percent or so above room air (room air has 21 percent oxygen), or 12 + 21 = 33 percent oxygen. There are some newer methods which some adults are finding more convenient and less noticeable to other people than the old methods. These include nasal cannulas which come through eyeglasses (and therefore have just a little bit of tubing sticking out the end of the eyeglass nosepiece), and oxygen through a tiny tracheostomy (a small hole placed surgically in the neck; this way, the tubing can go under the clothes, and the tracheostomy itself can be hidden under a turtleneck or scarf). Other methods include oxygen tents, which surround the whole upper body; oxygen hoods, which surround the whole head; and single nasal tubes (with one thin tube going into the nostril). Most of these last methods are useful mainly for babies, and therefore are not used very much in CF, since babies with CF usually don't need extra oxygen.

Amount needed: Your doctor may want to do a "blood gas" to see how much oxygen you have in your blood before he or she decides whether you need extra oxygen. This test involves taking blood from an artery (usually the radial artery, at the wrist), and is therefore somewhat more painful than most blood tests, which are usually taken from a vein (closer to the skin surface than arteries). However, if some lidocaine or other local anesthetic is used, this is not a painful test, and it can be very important. To understand how much extra oxygen is needed, you have to understand how the brain directs breathing. This is discussed in Chapter 1: *The Respiratory System.*

Undesirable effects: The main danger of oxygen is giving so much that it turns off the signal to breathe. Oxygen is also very dry, even when it's been humidified (as it should always be before it's breathed), and can make the mouth and nose uncomfortably dry. Too much oxygen can be toxic to lung tissue (this is not a problem with less than 40 percent oxygen). The problem you might have heard of concerning eye damage from oxygen is only true in premature babies.

Addiction: Some people worry that once they start on oxygen they'll become addicted in the way that someone gets addicted to morphine or heroin. This does not happen. People whose lungs are bad enough that they need extra oxygen feel much better when they take that oxygen, and they won't want to stop taking it while their lungs are still in that condition. But if the lung disease improves, and extra oxygen is not needed any more, people don't continue to desire the extra oxygen because the body is now supplying it. If the lungs cannot improve, the person will continue to want to use the oxygen, but this is not an addiction.

Cough Medicines

There are two main kinds of medicines which usually are referred to as "cough medicines." One of these is the expectorants. Expectorants are intended to make it easier to bring up mucus from the lungs. This is a good idea, but unfortunately these drugs don't work. The other kind of cough medicine is the cough suppressant, that is, a drug which controls the cough center in the brain, and says, "don't cough, no matter what is in the lungs that needs to come up." This is usually a terrible idea, especially for someone with CF. Some drug preparations are available which combine these two types of cough medicine, which have opposite goals! In the majority of cases, including most patients with CF, cough is an important defense mechanism which keeps the lungs clear of substances that shouldn't be there. Cough is a sign that something is wrong, but efforts should be directed at what is wrong. If someone is coughing because of bronchospasm, a bronchodilator will relieve the bronchospasm, and thus stop the cough; in a sense, it is a good kind of cough medicine. Similarly, if someone with CF is coughing because infection in the bronchi has gotten out of control, antibiotics are probably needed; they may control the infection and thus stop the cough. Other kinds of cough medicines are rarely very useful.

Upper Airway

Polyp Medicines

Many people with CF have nasal polyps, which are growths of extra tissue (not cancer) in the nose. Usually these cause no problems except mild stuffiness, but they can get large enough to be seen at the end of the nose or block one side of the nose so you can't breathe through it. A few medicines have been used to shrink polyps, and some people feel that they work. These medicines include antihistamines, decongestants (like Neo-Synephrine), and steroid sprays (like Beconase, Vancenase, and Nasalide). A person with nasal allergy symptoms may also be helped by some of these same nasal sprays.

Sinus Medicines

On X-ray examination, most CF patients appear to have abnormal sinuses. Usually this bothers the radiologist more than the patient. Occasionally, there can be actual sinus infection (sinusitis) which may be a nuisance to the patient. In these cases, doctors may prescribe a decongestant and/or antibiotics.

Allergies

Allergies can cause problems with either the upper respiratory system (stuffy sneezy nose) or lungs (congestion, wheezing) or both. CF patients are somewhat more likely than people without CF to have allergies. It is often very difficult to tell if an upper or lower airway problem is caused by infection or by allergy. Complicating the matter is that either one can probably make the other worse, so that constriction of the bronchi from a pollen allergy will make it harder to clear mucus from the bronchi, and make it easier for infection to get out of control.

Antihistamines

Histamine is a chemical that is released from white blood cells in response to different things including irritation and allergy. Its release can cause many of the problems we associate with allergies: runny nose, itchy nose, constricted bronchi, hives. Antihistamines do not stop the release of histamine from the blood cells, but they do help to block its action in the nose, skin, etc.

How taken: These are most commonly taken by mouth but can be given by injection.

Undesirable effects: The most common and often the most troublesome side effect from these drugs is drowsiness. They can also cause a dry mouth.

Decongestants

These drugs are supposed to make the nose less stuffy. Although they are used by milions of people, there is not very much scientific evidence that they work.

Allergy Shots

This is a very controversial topic. Most pulmonary specialists feel that allergy shots may be helpful for nasal allergies but not for bronchial allergies (asthma), while many allergists feel that they sometimes can be helpful for asthma too. There is nothing about CF which makes someone more or less likely to respond well to allergy shots than anyone else.

The Heart

The heart is not directly affected by CF, and most people with CF have very good hearts. Therefore, there usually is no need of heart medications. However, if someone's lungs become badly diseased (from CF or any other cause), the heart may not be able to pump all the necessary fluid through the diseased lungs. When this happens, two types of medicines are sometimes used: diuretics and digitalis.

Diuretics

These drugs help the kidneys get rid of extra fluid that may have built up in the body because of the heart's inability to pump all of the fluid. Most doctors agree that when someone has heart failure because of severe lung disease, it is very important to cut down on the amount of fluid that the heart is asked to pump. This is accomplished through restricting the amount of salt and fluid consumed and through careful use of diuretic medicines.

Furosemide

How taken: Furosemide (Lasix) can be taken by mouth (tablet, liquid) or by injection (either IM or IV).

Undesirable effects: Furosemide causes the body to lose potassium in addition to other salts and this can upset the body's salt balance if used in high doses every day for too long. This effect can be lessened by an every-other-day schedule in people who tolerate this schedule. The drug can also do too much of a good thing—in eliminating too much excess fluid, it may actually dehydrate the patient. Furosemide has been associated with some cases of hearing problems, which are usually reversible. Occasionally, someone who is allergic to sulfa drugs may be allergic to furosemide.

Spironolactone (Aldactone)

This drug is less powerful than furosemide, but keeps the body from losing potassium.

How taken: oral tablets.

Undesirable effects: Any diuretic may cause excess loss of water (dehydration) and salt balance problems. Spironolactone may also give some GI upset. A rash is sometimes seen. It may cause breast enlargement and/or impotence in men. These effects are nearly always temporary and disappear when the drug is stopped.

Thiazides

How taken: These diuretics are usually taken by mouth (tablet; although a liquid preparation is also available). Rarely they may be given by IV, but not by IM injection.

Undesirable effects: These are quite safe and usually there are no problems. Textbooks do list many possible reactions, including GI upset, dizziness, fatigue, headache, anemia, weakness, muscle spasms, gout.

Digitalis

This drug has been known for centuries and is very effective in making the heart contractions stronger. It is not clear whether it is helpful in people whose heart problems are mainly caused by lung problems.

How taken: Digitalis preparations can be taken by mouth (tablets or liquids) or by IV injection.

Undesirable effects: Too much digitalis can be very dangerous and can cause heart beat irregularities, confusion, visual problems, vomiting, diarrhea, headache, weakness.

GASTROINTESTINAL AND DIGESTIVE SYSTEM MEDICATIONS

The main problem in the gastrointestinal and digestive system is the thick mucus that blocks the ducts of the pancreas and prevents the digestive chemicals ("enzymes") from reaching the intestines where they mix with the food that has been eaten. If these digestive enzymes are not available, the food cannot be digested, that is, broken down into particles small enough to be soaked up into the bloodstream through the wall of the intestine. As a result, a lot of the food (especially the fat) will not be available to the body and will pass out into the stools. Most (but not all) CF patients have this problem. Another gastrointestinal problem is that the intestines' own mucus is very thick which can sometimes lead to blockage of the intestines.

Digestive Enzymes

These enzymes come from the pancreas of animals. They have changed what used to be a serious, even fatal, problem into a nuisance problem. With enzyme type and dosage properly adjusted, most CF patients are able to absorb the majority of what they eat (even the fat). Thus, they are able to get the nutritional value from the food which would be lost without the enzymes.

Types of Enzymes

"REGULAR" ENZYMES. These enzymes (such as Viokase and Cotazym) have served CF patients very well for many years. They were available in powders, capsules

(Cotazym), or tablets (Viokase). They are seldom used now because the enteric-coated enzymes are usually more effective.

"REGULAR" PLUS BILE SALTS. Bile salts are necessary for complete digestion and absorption of food, and CF patients may have low levels of bile salts. There are a few preparations available which combine enzymes and bile salts. These are probably not needed by most patients.

ENTERIC-COATED. These enzymes come in capsules with little coated beads inside. The coating protects the enzyme inside each bead so that it is not destroyed by stomach acid. The coating is designed to dissolve once the beads are past the stomach and are in the intestine, where these enzymes are supposed to do their work. This protection of the enzymes from the destructive influence of stomach acid has brought about a huge improvement in the effectiveness of enzymes for most patients with CF.

Method of Taking Enzymes

Enzymes work by mixing with the food and digesting it. Normally, this is supposed to happen in the duodenum. Duplicating this process requires taking the enzymes by mouth, at mealtime. Thus, this is not a once-a-day or three-times-a-day kind of medicine. When you're not eating, you don't need to take enzymes, and when you eat five times a day, you need enzymes five times. This is particularly true for fat and protein, and less so for carbohydrates (so if you're just having a soft drink or sugar candy, you don't need to take enzymes). Anyone old enough to swallow capsules can just swallow enzyme capsules as they eat. Some doctors advise taking all the enzymes at the beginning of the meal, while others prefer one-half at the beginning and one-half part way through the meal. Babies who can't swallow whole capsules can still use enzymes—just empty the capsule into some applesauce or other soft food. Even the smallest babies, who are not yet on solids, can use these enzymes if you put the beads in the baby's mouth, then give a bottle to wash them down.

How Much to Take?

This is difficult to answer precisely, but the needed amount can be easily estimated. This is yet another area where common sense can enable patients and families to figure out the best way to do things. The main thing to keep in mind is that the more food (especially fat) that goes in the mouth, the more enzymes are needed to process it. There's a built-in enzymemeter: if there is not enough enzyme to digest the fat, what isn't digested will come out in the stool, making the stools larger, greasier, less formed, more frequent, more likely to float, and with a stronger odor. Therefore, it's usually easy to check the results in the bathroom. If there is too much fat coming out in the stool, you need to adjust the amount of enzyme. You will soon learn that certain meals demand more enzymes than others (pizza and chili are special offenders). You can adjust the enzyme dosage to match the diet. However, don't make drastic changes in enzymes just because of one "messy" stool; instead, make sure there's a pattern. Also remember that too much fat in the stool means not enough enzymes have been used for the amount of fat in the diet, so if you're adjusting the balance, you can cut down on the amount of fat you put in the diet, or add more enzymes. Since cutting down on the amount of fat in the diet will mean giving fewer calories which can help with growth and energy, etc., it's usually best to add more enzymes. Newer enzyme preparations can give you up to 4 times as much enzyme activity in the same size capsule. (See the table under *Enzymes* in the *Glossary of Drugs* at the end of Appendix B.)

Anti-Acid Drugs

Excess stomach acid can cause several different types of problems in anyone, and at least one additional problem if someone has CF. Too much acid can destroy the old kind of digestive enzyme medicines, although this is much less a problem with enteric-coated enzymes. Too much acid can also help cause ulcers. Occasionally, the stomach acid can reflux (go backwards) up into the esophagus causing heartburn (the burning discomfort felt when the esophagus becomes irritated from acid). Drugs that prevent the stomach from making too much acid, or drugs which neutralize the acid once it is made, may be helpful for any of these problems.

Cimetidine

Cimetidine (Tagemet) is now one of the most prescribed drugs in the world, largely because it is very effective in decreasing the production of stomach acid.

How taken: Cimetidine is almost always taken by mouth, in a tablet, or liquid, usually before meals and before bed.

Undesirable effects: This is a fairly new drug so it is possible that new problems will be discovered. For now it seems to be relatively safe. Mild diarrhea, headache, or swelling of breasts have been seen in people taking cimetidine, but none of these problems is common.

Ranitidine

Ranitidine (Zantac) is a close relative of cimetidine, and is an even newer drug. It can be taken at a lower dose, less frequently, with comparable effects to cimetidine.

Various Antacids

These medicines, taken by mouth as chewable tablets or the more effective liquid form, do not influence how much acid is produced by the stomach, but they can neutralize the acid once it's formed.

Anticonstipation Medicines

Constipation is seldom a problem in patients with CF, but it does occur occasionally. Failure to pass any stool can be an important sign of a dangerous intestinal obstruction called meconium ileus in newborn infant and meconium ileus equivalent in someone older.

Dietary Fiber

Someone who has difficulty passing bowel movements may benefit from increasing the amount of fiber in the diet. Foods high in fiber include fruits and some vegetables; bran is an especially good source of fiber. Breakfast cereals with bran should have at least 4 grams (gm) of dietary fiber per serving to be effective (this information is included on the side-panel of the cereal box; if the information isn't there, it's likely that there is very little fiber in the cereal).

Enzymes

Before more drastic measures are undertaken, it usually helps to make sure the digestive enzyme dose is appropriate, since very bulky poorly digested stools may make blockage more likely.

Mineral Oil

On some occasions a physician may prescribe oral mineral oil to help pass stools.

Bowel Stimulants

If someone is not completely blocked up, some medications which stimulate intestinal contractions may help the bowels to empty. Senekot is one such laxative.

Enemas

With more blockage, enemas may be needed to help wash out the lower intestines. Generally, several types of enemas can be used in different situations. Always check with your doctor to be sure it's safe to use an enema, and to find out which kind.

GASTROGRAFIN ENEMAS. Severe intestinal obstruction is a serious matter that used to be treatable only with surgery. Fortunately today, many cases can be treated in the hospital with special enemas. Gastrografin is a substance which can be used for an enema, and has several useful properties. It shows up on X-ray, so the radiologist can see the outline of the bowel to make sure there is not another problem causing intestinal blockage, and to make sure the enema is going far up into the intestines so that it will work. It's very slippery, allowing it to slip by the blockage. It also acts like a sponge, pulling in lots of fluid from the rest of the body to help make the stools stuck in the bowel become more watery and easier to move out.

How performed: These enemas always must be done where there is X-ray equipment and a radiologist. This usually means they are done in the hospital. Most children who need them are sick enough to need to be in the hospital anyway.

Undesirable effects: These enemas are somewhat uncomfortable, as is true of any enema, but they can provide prompt relief from the abdominal pain from intestinal blockage. The main danger of this procedure is that so much fluid is pulled into the bowel from the rest of the body that the patient can become dehydrated. For this reason, most doctors will not perform this procedure on an infant unless the baby has an IV line in place, with fluids running in.

Miscellaneous

1. GOLYTELY. A salty liquid which can be drunk in large quantities to "Flush out" the intestines.

2. COLACE. A stool softener.

3. LACTULOSE (CEFULAC, CHRONULAC). A medicine taken by mouth which pulls fluid into the intestines to help make the bowel contents more watery, and easier to move.

Antibloating Medications

Some patients with CF have trouble with abdominal bloating. This may be caused by the thick mucus in the intestines which can surround little air bubbles which does not let the little bubbles get together to make a single bubble that is big enough for a burp. Some drugs containing simethicone (Mylicon, Silain) may help dissolve some of that mucus and allow a gentle upwards or downwards explosion of that air, relieving the pressure and discomfort. These drugs are taken by mouth (tablets or drops) and are very safe.

Vitamins

These are not really drugs, and should be a regular part of the diet. Four vitamins (A, D, E, K) are "fat soluble," meaning that they dissolve in fat and are only absorbed in the body when fats are absorbed. Thus, patients who have trouble absorbing fats may have low levels of these vitamins. For this reason, most nutrition experts agree that CF patients should probably receive supplements of these vitamins, at least some of the time. Vitamins A and D can probably be supplied from regular multivitamin preparations, but vitamin K and vitamin E need to be taken separately. For the vitamin E, most preparations you can buy will not work for someone who has trouble absorbing fats, and a form which is partly dissolvable in water needs to be used.

Growth and Appetite Stimulants and Supplements

Hormones

Most of the drugs used to stimulate appetite and growth are anabolic steroids and androgens (male hormones). They are widely used, but have not been conclusively shown to be safe or effective in patients with CF.

How taken: These hormones can be given by injection or taken by mouth.

Undesirable effects: These are too numerous to list completely, are worrisome, and can actually result in stopping growth sooner than it would have stopped naturally (as these hormones increase bone growth, they also close the growth plate of the bones—the part of the bones where growth takes place—more quickly than normal). Other undesirable effects include fluid retention, hirsutism (increased hairiness), baldness, various genital disturbances (too big, too little, too excitable, not excitable enough), acne, sleeplessness, liver disease, nausea, ulcer-like symptoms, and finally, disqualification from the Olympics.

Diet Supplements

Many different kinds of diet supplements are available, from vanilla milk shakes and ice cream sundaes to expensive "elemental" (predigested) formulas. These supplements usually have high amounts of calories. They seem to be helpful in some people, while in others, the number of calories taken in with the supplements is balanced by the number of calories not eaten in the regular meals. Some programs have been successful in helping patients gain weight and height by running nighttime feedings of these dietary supplements through a stomach-tube while the patients sleep. Such a program, of course, should never be undertaken without your doctor's knowledge and cooperation.

How taken: Some of these can be sprinkled on top of regular meals; some can be eaten between meals. Others are designed to be given through a tube (mostly because they taste so bad, but also because they can be given very slowly while the patient sleeps).

Undesirable effects: The supplements may interfere with normal mealtime appetite. The tube feedings require a tube which can be somewhat uncomfortable and/or inconvenient. Several tubes can be used, including a nasogastric tube, which goes through the nose ("naso-") into the stomach ("gastric"), and is usually put in each evening and removed in the morning. Another kind of tube is a permanent tube placed by a surgical operation which makes a hole or stoma in the wall of the abdomen directly into the stomach (a gastrostomy tube) or into the second part of the small intestine, the jejunum (a feeding jejunostomy tube). Possible problems from these nighttime feedings include overfilling the stomach.

GLOSSARY OF DRUGS

This glossary is a partial list of drugs, which can be found under both their generic and trade names. Drugs that are discussed in this appendix contain references to the appropriate section. For example, PenVee K is a form of the antibiotic, penicillin, which is discussed under **Lungs:** *Antibiotics: Penicillins,* on page 158.

Accelerase   (triacylglycerol lipase) A digestive enzyme with bile salts (*see* page 170).

Accurbron   A theophylline (*see* page 163).

acetylcysteine   A mucolytic (*see* page 165).

Actifed   (triprolidine hydrochloride + pseudoephedrine hydrochloride) A decongestant/antihistamine combination (*see* page 168).

Adrenalin   (epinephrine) A bronchodilator (*see* page 162).

Aerolate Jr. and Sr.   Theophylline bronchodilators (*see* page 163).

Afrin   (oxymetazoline hydrochloride) A decongestant (*see* page 168).

albuterol   A beta-agonist bronchodilator (*see* page 163).

Aldactone   (spironolactone) A diuretic (*see* page 169).

Allerest   A decongestant/antihistamine (*see* page 168).

amantadine hydrochloride   A medication that can help control infection with the influenza virus.

Amcill   (ampicillin) An antibiotic (*see* page 158).

amikacin sulfate   An aminoglycoside antibiotic (*see* page 157).

Amikin   Amikacin sulfate, an aminoglycoside (*see* page 157).

Aminodur   A theophylline bronchodilator (*see* page 163).

aminophylline   A theophylline bronchodilator (*see* page 163).

amoxicillin   An antibiotic (*see* page 158).

Amoxil   Amoxicillin (*see* page 158).

Amphojel   (aluminum hydroxide gel) An antacid (*see* page 172).

ampicillin   An antibiotic; an effective antibacterial agent (*see* page 158).

Ancef   (cefazolin sodium) A cephalosporin antibiotic (*see* page 161).

Aquasol A   A vitamin A preparation (*see* page 174).

Aquasol E   A vitamin E preparation (*see* page 174).

Asbron   A theophylline bronchodilator (*see* page 163).

Atuss   A cough medicine that includes a cough-suppressant, an antihistamine, and a decongestant (*see* page 167).

Augmentin   (amoxicillin/clavulanate potassium) An antibiotic (*see* page 158).

Avazyme   (chymotrypsin) A digestive enzyme, useful only for digesting protein, and not fat (*see* page 170).

Azactam   (*see* Aztreonam *below*).

azlocillin   An anti-*Pseudomonas* antibiotic (*see* page 159).

Azmacort   (triamcinolone acetonide) An inhaled corticosteroid (*see* page 164).

aztreonam   An anti-*Pseudomonas* antibiotic (*see* page 162).

bacampicillin HCl   An ampicillin (*see* page 158).

Bactrim   (trimethoprim-sulfamethoxazole) A combination antibiotic (*see* page 157).

Bactrim DS   Double-strength Bactrim (*see* Bactrim).

Basaljel   (aluminum carbonate gel) An antacid (*see* page 172).

beclomethasone dipropionate   An inhaled corticosteroid (*see* page 164).

Beclovent   (beclomethasone dipropionate) A corticosteroid (*see* page 164).

Beconase   (beclomethasone dipropionate) A nasal steroid spray often used for polyps or nasal allergies (*see* page 164).

Beepen-VK   (penicillin) An antibiotic (*see* page 158).

Benadryl   (diphenhydramine hydrochloride) An antihistamine (*see* page 168).

Betapen-VK   (penicillin V potassium) An antibiotic (*see* page 158).

Bicillin   (penicillin G benzathine) An injectable (IM) penicillin (*see* page 158).

Bilezyme   A digestive enzyme combination containing protein-digesting enzymes but no fat-digesting enzymes. Also contains bile salts (*see* page 171).

Bilogen   A digestive enzyme that contains protein-digesting enzymes but no fat-digesting enzymes. Also contains bile salts (*see* page 171).

bisacodyl   A laxative (*see* page 172).

bran   A very rich source of dietary fiber. Taken in pure form, it tastes like rabbit food, but is very effective (*see* page 173).

Brethine   (terbutaline sulfate) A beta-agonist bronchodilator (*see* page 163).

Bricanyl   (terbutaline sulfate) A beta-agonist bronchodilator (*see* page 163).

Bristagen   (gentamicin) An aminoglycoside antibiotic (*see* page 159).

Bristamycin   An erythromycin (stearate) antibiotic (*see* page 161).

Bronchobid Duracaps   A combination bronchodilator drug that includes theophylline and ephedrine, related to the beta-agonists (*see* page 163).

Broncholate Capsules   A combination bronchodilator including theophylline and ephedrine (*See* Bronchobid *above*).

Brondecon   (oxtriphylline + guaifenesin) A bronchodilator and "expectorant" combination. The bronchodilator is oxtriphylline, a close relative of theophylline (*see* page 162). The expectorant is called guaifenesin (*see* page 167).

Brondelate   Same as Brondecon.

Bronitin Mist   An adrenaline inhaler.

Bronkaid   A strong bronchodilator that contains theophylline (*see* page 163), guaifenesin, and expectorant (*see* page 167).

Bronkaid Mist   An adrenaline inhaler.

Bronkodyl   A theophylline (*see* page 163).

Bronkolixir A combination bronchodilator that contains theophylline, ephedrine sulfate (related to beta-agonists) (*see* page 163), guaifenesin, an expectorant (*see* page 167), and phenobarbital. Phenobarbital is a potent sedative whose proper use is in people with psychiatric illness to control agitation, anxiety, and insomnia, and as a seizure medication in patients who have epilepsy. It is useless as a bronchodilator. (In this particular preparation, all of the medications are in such low dose that they do neither good nor harm anyway.)

Bronkometer (isoetharine mesylate) A form of a beta$_2$-bronchodilator for inhalation (*see* page 163).

Bronkosol (isoetharine HCl) A beta-agonist bronchodilator, for use in an aerosol (*see* page 162).

Bronkotabs A combination theophylline bronchodilator, ephedrine (*see* page 162), guaifenesin (*see* page 167), and phenobarbital (*see* Broncholixir).

carbenicillin An anti-*Pseudomonas* antibiotic (*see* page 159).

Ceclor (cefaclor) A cephalosporin antibiotic (*see* page 161).

cefaclor A cephalosporin antibiotic (*see* page 161).

cefadroxil A cephalosporin antibiotic (*see* page 161).

Cefadyl (cephapirin sodium) A cephalosporin antibiotic (*see* page 161).

cefamandole A cephalosporin antibiotic (*see* page 161).

cefazolin An analogue of a cephalosporin antibiotic (*see* page 161).

Cefobid A cephalosporin antibiotic with some effect against *Pseudomonas*.

cefoperozone A cephalosporin antibiotic with some effect against *Pseudomonas*.

cefotaxime A cephalosporin antibiotic (*see* page 161).

cefoxitin An analogue derivative of a cephalosporin antibiotic (*see* page 161).

ceftazidime An anti-*Pseudomonas* cephalosporin (*see* page 161).

Cefulac (lactulose) An anticonstipation medication (*see* page 172).

Celbenin (sodium methicillin) An anti-*Staph* antibiotic (*see* page 158).

Cenalax An anticonstipation drug (*see* page 172).

cephalexin A cephalosporin antibiotic (*see* page 161).

cephaloglycin A cephalosporin antibiotic (*see* page 161).

cephaloridine A cephalosporin antibiotic (*see* page 161).

cephalosporins A family of antibiotics (*see* page 161).

cephalothin A cephalosporin antibiotic (*see* page 161).

cephapirin A cephalosporin antibiotic (*see* page 161).

cephradine A cephalosporin antibiotic (*see* page 161).

Cerose A combination of various cough medicines (*see* page 167).

Cerylin A combination theophylline bronchodilator (*see* page 163) and guaifenesin expectorant (*see* page 167).

chloramphenicol An antibiotic (*see* page 160).

Chloromycetin (chloramphenicol) An antibiotic.

Chlor-Trimeton (pseudoephedrine sulfate + chlorpheniramine maleate) An antihistamine (*see* page 168).

Choledyl (oxtriphylline) A bronchodilator closely related to theophylline (*see* page 163).

cimetidine An antacid preparation (*see* page 172).

Cipro A quinolone antibiotic.

ciprofloxacin A quinolone antibiotic (*see* page 161).

Claforan A cephalosporin antibiotic (*see* page 161).

Cleocin (clindamycin) One of the aminoglycoside antibiotics (*see* page 159).

clindamycin An aminoglycoside antibiotic (*see* page 159).

cloxacillin An anti-*Staph* penicillin (*see* page 159).

Cloxapen (cloxacillin) A penicillin.

codeine A cough suppressant (*see* page 167).

cod liver oil A traditional source of vitamins A and D whose main advantage is its bad taste (*see* page 174).

coffee A caffeine-containing popular drink. Caffeine is also found in Coca-Cola, Pepsi, and in some cases serves as a bronchodilator (*see* page 162).

Colace (docusate sodium) A stool softener (*see* page 174).

colistin A very potent antibiotic, a relative of the aminoglycosides. Given intravenously it can have severe side effects including headaches and kidney damage (*see* page 159).

Coly-Mycin S (colistin sulfate) An antibiotic.

Contac An antihistamine and decongestant (*see* page 168).

Co-Pyronil (pyrrobutamine compound) An antihistamine and decongestant combination (*see* page 168).

Coricidin An antihistamine and decongestant.

Cotazym (pancrelipase) A pancreatic digestive enzyme (*see* page 170 and Table 1, page 182).

Cotazym-B A digestive enzyme with bile salts (*see* page 170).

Cotazym-S An enteric-coated pancreatic enzyme (*see* page 171 and Table 1, page 182).

co-trimoxazole A combination antibiotic (trimethoprim-sulfamethoxazole) (*see* page 159).

Co-Tylenol A combination of decongestant, antihistamine, and cough suppressant with acetaminophen (*see* pages 167 and 168).

Creon (pancreatin) An enteric-coated pancreatic enzyme (*see* page 171).

Criticare A nutritional supplement and formula that is very low in fat and whose protein is predigested (*see* page 175).

cromolyn   An inhaled medicine used to prevent bronchospasm (*see* page 162).

cyclacillin   "Twin brother" of ampicillin; an effective antibacterial agent (*see* page 158).

Cyclapen   (cyclacillin) (*see* page 158).

Decadron   (dexamethasone) A steroid (*see* page 164).

Declomycin   (demeclocycline) A tetracycline antibiotic (*see* page 161).

Delatestryl   (testosterone enanthate) A male hormone sometimes used to stimulate growth and appetite (*see* page 174).

Deltasone   (prednisone) A steroid sometimes used to decrease bronchial inflammation (*see* page 164).

Demazin   (chlorpheniramine maleate + phenylephine hydrochloride) A combination antihistamine-decongestant (*see* pages 167 and 168).

demeclocycline   A tetracycline antibiotic (*see* page 161).

Demerol   (meperidine [pethidine] hydrochloride) A narcotic painkiller and sedative.

Depo-Testosterone   A male hormone (testosterone) in injectable form sometimes used as a growth and appetite stimulant (*see* page 174).

De-Tuss   A combination cough medicine and antihistamine (*see* page 168).

dexamethasone   A steroid that is sometimes taken by aerosol inhalation (*see* page 164).

dextromethorphan (DM)   A cough suppressant (*see* page 167).

Dianabol   (methandrostenolone) An anabolic and male sex hormone sometimes used for growth and appetite stimulant (*see* page 174).

dicloxacillin sodium   An anti-*Staph* penicillin (*see* page 159).

digitalis   A drug that strengthens heart contractions (*see* page 170).

digitoxin   A digitalis drug (*see* page 170).

digoxin   A digitalis drug (*see* page 170).

Dilaudid   (hydromorphone hydrochloride) A narcotic that is occasionally used for pain and for cough suppression.

Dimetane   (brompheniramine maleate) A combination cough medicine, antihistamine, and decongestant (*see* page 167).

Dimetapp   Similar to Dimetane.

diphenhydramine hydrochloride   An antihistamine (*see* page 168).

disodium cromoglycate   crolyn; used in treatment of bronchial asthmas (*see* page 164).

diuretics   Medications that increase the kidneys' production of urine, and thus help rid the body of excess fluid (*see* page 169).

Donatussin   (chlorpheniramine maleate + phenylephrine hydrochloride + guaifenesin) A combination cough medicine, antihistamine, and decongestant.

Dorcol   (guaifenesin + phenylpropanolamine hydrochloride + dextromethorphan hydrobromide) A cough medicine that includes a decongestant and a cough suppressant (*see* page 167).

doxycycline A tetracycline antibiotic (*see* page 161).

Dristan A decongestant (*see* page 168).

Dynapen (dicloxacillin) An anti-*Staph* antibiotic (*see* page 159).

dyphylline A form of theophylline bronchodilator (*see* page 163).

EES (erythromycin ethylsuccinate) An erythromycin antibiotic (*see* page 161).

Elixicon (theophylline) A theophylline bronchodilator (*see* page 163).

Elixophyllin A form of theophylline bronchodilator (*see* page 163).

E-Mycin An erythromycin antibiotic (*see* page 161).

Ensure A calorie supplement (*see* page 175).

Entolase An enteric-coated digestive enzyme (*see* page 171 and Table 1, page 182).

Entolase-HP An enteric-coated digestive enzyme (*see* page 171 and Table 1, page 182).

enzymes Catalysts of chemical reactions; *see* Table 1 on next page (*see* page 170).

ephedrine Sometimes used as a bronchodilator (*see* page 162).

epinephrine Adrenalin. Often used as an emergency bronchodilator, similar in some of its action to the "beta-agonists" (*see* page 163), but with more effect on the heart (speeds it up).

Erythrocin An erythromycin antibiotic (*see* page 161).

erythromycin A family of antibiotics (*see* page 161).

ethacrynic acid A diuretic (*see* page 169).

fiber An important component of the diet (*see* page 173).

Fleet enemas Occasionally used for treating constipation (*see* page 173).

Fortaz (ceftazidime) A cephalosporin antibiotic (*see* page 161).

furosemide A diuretic (*see* page 169).

Gantrisin (sulfisoxazole) A sulfa antibiotic (*see* page 159).

Garamycin (gentamicin) An aminoglycoside antibiotic (*see* page 159).

Gastrografin (meglumine diatrizoate) A substance that is occasionally used in the hospital for an enema (*see* page 173).

Gaviscon (aluminum hydroxide + magnesium carbonate) An antacid (*see* page 172).

Gelusil (aluminum hydroxide + magnesium hydroxide + simethicone) An antacid (*see* page 172).

gentamicin An aminoglycoside antibiotic (*see* page 159).

Geocillin An oral form of the antibiotic carbenicillin. The oral form of the medicine is not effective for lung disease (*see* page 159).

Geopen An injectable form of carbenicillin (*see* page 159).

GoLYTELY A salty liquid which can be drunk in large quantities to "flush out" the intestines (*see* page 174).

TABLE 1. *Pancreatic enzymes*

Product	Manufacturer	Lipase[a]	Protease[b]	Amylase[c]	Special features
Cotazym	Organon	8,000	3,000	3,000	Capsules, cherry flavor, no enteric coating
Cotazym S	Organon	5,000	20,000	20,000	Capsules with enteric-coated spheres
Creon	Reid-Rowell	8,000	13,000	30,000	Brown and yellow capsules with enteric-coated spheres
Entolase	AH Robins	4,000	25,000	20,000	Enteric-coated, dye-free capsules
Entolase HP	AH Robins	8,000	50,000	40,000	Enteric-coated, dye-free capsules
Pancrease	McNeil	4,000	25,000	20,000	Dye-free; enteric-coated spheres in capsules
Pancrease MT4	McNeil	4,000	12,000	12,000	Dye-free; enteric-coated microtablets in very small capsules
Pancrease MT10	McNeil	10,000	30,000	30,000	Dye-free; enteric-coated microtablets in small capsules
Pancrease MT16	McNeil	16,000	48,000	48,000	Dye-free; enteric-coated microtablets in capsules
Pancreatin	Vitaline	12,000	60,000	60,000	Uncoated, buffered tablet
Viokase Tablet	Robins	8,000	30,000	30,000	No enteric coating
Viokase Powder	Robins	16,800	70,000	70,000	Amount per 1/4 teasp., no enteric coating
Zymase	Organon	12,000	24,000	24,000	Enteric-coated spheres in capsules

[a]Lipase, fat-digesting enzyme; most important for CF patients; one capsule with 8,000 units of lipase is roughly equivalent to two 4,000 unit-capsules of lipase (if all are enteric-coated or all non-enteric-coated).
[b]Protease, protein-digesting enzyme.
[c]Amylase, starch-digesting enzyme.
Numbers refer to content in international units.

Halotestin (fluoxymesterone) A male sex hormone sometimes used for growth and appetite stimulation (*see* page 174).

heparin An anticoagulant, that is, a drug which prevents clotting of the blood. This is very useful when used in very small amounts in a needle in a vein. It can keep the blood from clotting up the needle so that the needle can be used for a long time for administration of IV antibiotics.

heparin lock A needle which is inserted in the vein and periodically rinsed out with heparin solution. This enables the needle to be used for administration of intravenous antibiotics on an intermittent basis. Once rinsed out, the needle can be plugged up and just taped to the arm without any extra tubing connected to it, leaving the arm free.

Hep-Lock The dilute heparin solution used in a heparin lock.

hetacillin An antibiotic related to ampicillin (*see* page 158).

Hexadrol (dexamethasone) A steroid sometimes used to decrease bronchial inflammation (*see* page 164).

Hycodan (hydrocodone bitartrate) A combination cough medicine that contains a cough suppressant (*see* page 167).

Hycotuss (hydrocodone bitartrate + guaifenesin) A multiingredient cough medicine which includes a cough suppressant (*see* page 167).

hydrocodone bitartrate A narcotic sometimes used as a cough suppressant (*see* page 167).

hydrocortisone A steroid occasionally used in different forms to decrease bronchial inflammation (*see* page 164).

Ilozyme (pancrelipase) A pancreatic enzyme (*see* page 170).

imipenem An anti-*Pseudomonas* antibiotic (*see* page 161).

Intal cromolyn sodium (*see* page 164).

ipecac A medicine used to induce vomiting (usually used after a child has accidentally ingested a poisonous substance).

isoetharine A bronchodilator drug taken by inhalation (*see* page 162).

isoproterenol An inhaled bronchodilator (*see* page 162).

Isuprel (isoproterenol) A bronchodilator taken by inhalation (*see* page 162).

kanamycin An aminoglycoside antibiotic (*see* page 159).

Kantrex (kanamycin) An antibiotic (*see* page 159).

Keflex (cephalexin) A cephalosporin antibiotic (*see* page 161).

Keflin (cephalothin sodium) A cephalosporin antibiotic (*see* page 161).

Kefzol (cefazolin sodium) A cephalosporin antibiotic (*see* page 161).

lactulose An anticonstipation medication (*see* page 174).

Lanophyllin A form of theophylline bronchodilator (*see* page 163).

Lanoxin (digoxin) A type of digitalis (*see* page 170).

Larotid (amoxicillin) An antibiotic (*see* page 158).

Lasix (furosemide) A diuretic (*see* page 169).

Ledercillin   (penicillin G procaine) A form of penicillin (*see* page 158).

Lincocin   (lincomycin HCl) An antibiotic (*see* page 157).

lincomycin   An antibiotic not commonly used in CF (*see* page 157).

Lufyllin   (dyphylline) A theophylline bronchodilator (*see* page 163).

Maalox   An antacid (*see* page 172).

Marax   (ephedrine sulfate + theophylline + hydroxyzine HCl) A combination drug including a theophylline bronchodilator (*see* page 163) and another bronchodilator.

Medihaler-EPI   An inhaled form of epinephrine or adrenalin (*see* page 163).

Medihaler-ISO   (isoproterenol sulfate) An inhaled bronchodilator with isoproterenol (*see* page 163).

Metaprel   (metaproterenol sulfate) A beta-agonist bronchodilator (*see* page 163).

metaproterenol sulfate   A beta-agonist bronchodilator (*see* page 163).

methacycline   A tetracycline antibiotic (*see* page 161).

methicillin sulfate   An anti-*Staph* antibiotic (*see* page 158).

methyltestosterone   A male sex hormone, sometimes used as a growth and appetite stimulant (*see* page 174).

metoclopramide   A drug that increases the movement of foods through the gastrointestinal tract and which may decrease gastroesophageal reflux (*see* page 172).

Mezlin   (mezlocillin) An anti-*Pseudomonas* antibiotic (*see* page 161).

milk of magnesia   There are several different preparations: antacids (*see* page 172), and laxatives which are used as an anticonstipation preparation (*see* page 173).

Minocin   (minocycline HCl) An antibiotic (*see* page 157).

minocycline   A tetracycline antibiotic (*see* page 161).

mucolytics   Chemicals that break up mucus (*see* page 165).

Mucomyst   (acetylcysteine) A mucolytic (*see* page 165).

Mycostatin   (nystatin) A drug that kills yeast infections, which can appear when a patient is taking antibiotics. Mycostatin is occasionally prescribed when a child is taking antibiotics.

Mylanta   (aluminum hydroxide + magnesium hydroxide + simethicone) An antacid (*see* page 172).

Mylicon   (simethicone) An antibloating drug (*see* page 174).

Nafcil   (nafcillin sodium) An antibiotic.

nafcillin   An anti-*Staph* antibiotic (*see* page 158).

Naldecon   A decongestant antihistamine combination (*see* page 168).

Nebcin   (tobramycin sulfate) An aminoglycoside antibiotic (*see* page 159).

neomycin   An aminoglycoside antibiotic (*see* page 159).

Neo-Synephrine   (phenylephrine HCl) A decongestant (*see* page 168).

netilmicin   An aminoglycoside antibiotic (*see* page 159).

Novahistine   A combination of many ingredients, used for coughs and cold symptoms (*see* pages 167 and 168).

nystatin   Used to fight yeast infections which can appear when a patient is taking antibiotics.

Omnipen   (ampicillin) An antibiotic (*see* page 158).

Organidin   (iodinated glycerol) An expectorant (*see* page 167).

oxacillin   An anti-*Staph* antibiotic (*see* page 158).

oxtriphylline   A theophylline bronchodilator (*see* page 163).

oxytetracycline   A tetracycline antibiotic (*see* page 161).

Pancrease   (pancrelipase) An enteric-coated digestive enzyme (*see* page 171 and Table 1, page 182).

pancreatin   A digestive enzyme (*see* page 170 and Table 1, page 182).

pancrelipase   A digestive enzyme (*see* page 170).

Panmycin   (tetracycline) An antibiotic (*see* page 161).

Papase   A drug with some enzyme activity (*see* page 170).

Pediamycin   (erythromycin ethylsuccinate) An erythromycin antibiotic (*see* page 161).

Pediazole   (erythromycin ethylsuccinate + sulfisoxazole acetyl) A combination antibiotic that contains erythromycin and a sulfa drug (*see* page 161).

penicillin   An antibiotic (*see* page 158).

Pen-Vee-K   A penicillin antibiotic (*see* page 158).

phenylephrine hydrochloride   A medication sometimes used in aerosols. It constricts blood vessels and may therefore cut down on swelling in the bronchi by decreasing the blood flow to the bronchi.

piperacillin sodium   An anti-*Pseudomonas* antibiotic (*see* page 161).

Pipracil   (piperacillin) An antibiotic.

Pneumovax   The so-called "pneumonia vaccine." This is useful for children who have a particular deficiency in their body defenses which enables them to become infected with a germ called pneumococcus, such as children with sickle-cell disease. Many physicians feel that it is of no particular value to patients with cystic fibrosis.

Polycillin   (ampicillin) An antibiotic (*see* page 158).

Polycose   A high calorie diet supplement (*see* page 175).

Poly-Histine   A cough and cold preparation (*see* page 167).

Polymox   (amoxicillin) An antibiotic (*see* page 158).

polymyxin-B   An antibiotic (*see* page 157).

polymyxin-E   An antibiotic, also known as colistin, that is effective against *Pseudomonas*; however, it is often difficult to tolerate (*see* page 161).

prednisolone   A steroid used to decrease bronchial inflammation (*see* page 164).

prednisone   A steroid used to decrease bronchial inflammation (*see* page 164).

Primaxin (imipenem) An antibiotic with some activity against *Pseudomonas* (*see* page 161).

Principen (ampicillin) An antibiotic (*see* page 158).

Prostaphlin (oxacillin sodium) An anti-*Staph* penicillin antibiotic (*see* page 158).

Proventil A beta-agonist bronchodilator (*see* page 163).

prunes One of the best sources of dietary fiber, especially effective in combatting constipation (*see* page 173).

Quibron A bronchodilator preparation that contains several different drugs, including theophylline and an expectorant (*see* page 163).

quinolones A family of antibiotics (*see* page 161).

ranitidine A medication that decreases the stomach's production of acid (*see* page 172).

Reglan (metoclopramide) (*see* page 172).

ribavirin An aerosol medicine which can help control some viral bronchial infections, especially bronchiolitis caused by RSV (respiratory syncytial virus).

Robitussin (guaifenesin) A cough preparation consisting of an expectorant (*see* page 167).

Rondec (carbinoxamine maleate + pseudoephedrine HCl) A cough and cold preparation (*see* page 167).

saline Salt water.

Senekot (senna) An intestinal stimulant (*see* page 173).

Silain (simethicone) An antibloating drug (*see* page 174).

Slo-Phyllin Gyrocaps A long-lasting theophylline bronchodilator (*see* page 163).

sodium chloride Salt.

Somophyllin A theophylline preparation (*see* page 163).

Spectrobid A type of penicillin closely related to ampicillin.

spironolactone A diuretic (*see* page 169).

Staphcillin (sodium methicillin) (*see* page 158).

steroids Very potent drugs which are similar to the chemicals made in the body in the adrenal glands. They are very powerful and can be used safely for a short period of time for some purposes such as decreasing bronchial inflammation (*see* page 162). They are often employed for other purposes too, including growth and appetite stimulation (*see* page 174).

sulfamethoxazole A sulfa antibiotic (*see* page 159).

Sulfatrim A combination antibiotic trimethoprim-sulfamethaxozole (*see* page 159).

Sus-Phrine (epinephrine) A bronchodilator medication with some beta-agonist activity. It is used only by injection, and primarily for treating serious allergic reactions or an asthma attack (*see* page 162).

Sustacal A nutritional supplement formula (*see* page 175).

Sustaire A theophylline bronchodilator (*see* page 163).

Tagamet (cimetidine) An anti-acid drug (*see* page 172).

Tazidime ceftazidime (*see* page 161).

Tedral A combination drug which includes some theophylline bronchodilator (*see* page 163).

Tegopen (cloxacillin sodium) An anti-*Staph* penicillin (*see* page 158).

terbutaline sulfate A beta-agonist bronchodilator (*see* page 163).

Terramycin (oxytetracycline) A tetracycline antibiotic (*see* page 161).

Testionate A male steroid hormone used for growth and appetite stimulation (*see* page 175).

testosterone The primary male hormone (*see* page 175).

Tetra-BID A tetracycline antibiotic (*see* page 161).

tetracycline An antibiotic family (*see* page 157).

Theobid A theophylline bronchodilator (*see* page 163).

Theo-Dur A theophylline bronchodilator (*see* page 163).

Theolate A theophylline bronchodilator (*see* page 163).

Theophyl A theophylline bronchodilator (*see* page 163).

theophylline A family of bronchodilators (*see* page 163).

Theospan A theophylline bronchodilator (*see* page 163).

ticarcillin An anti-*Pseudomonas* penicillin (*see* page 159).

Timentin An anti-*Pseudomonas* and anti-*Staph* antibiotic (*see* page 159).

tobramycin An aminoglycoside antibiotic (*see* page 159).

Tornalate (methanesulfonate) A beta-agonist bronchodilator (*see* page 163).

triamcinolone An inhaled steroid (*see* page 164).

Triaminic (phenylpropanolamine HCl + pheniramine maleate + pyrilamine maleate) A cold preparation (*see* page 168).

trimethoprim An antibiotic usually found in combination with a sulfa drug (*see* page 159).

Tussionex A cough mixture including an antihistamine, a narcotic cough suppressant (*see* page 167).

Tuss-Ornade A cough medicine which also contains a decongestant and a cough suppressant (*see* page 168).

Vancenase (beclomethasone dipropionate) A nasal steroid spray (*see* page 164).

Veetid B-Cillin (penicillin) An antibiotic (*see* page 158).

Velosef A cephalosporin antibiotic (*see* page 161).

Ventolin (albuterol sulfate) A beta-agonist bronchodilator (*see* page 163).

Vibramycin A tetracycline antibiotic (*see* page 161).

Viokase (pancreatin) A digestive enzyme (*see* page 173 and Table 1, page 182).

Vipep A nutritional supplement formula (*see* page 175).

Virazole (ribavirin).

Vital A nutritional supplement formula (*see* page 175).

Vivonex A nutritional supplement formula (*see* page 175).

Winstrol (stanozolol) A sex steroid hormone (*see* page 174).

Wycillin (penicillin) An antibiotic (*see* page 158).

Zantac (ranitidine) Helps to decrease the stomach's production of acid (*see* page 172).

Zymase A digestive enzyme (*see* page 173 and Table 1, page 182).

C// Postural Drainage Techniques[a]

INFANTS

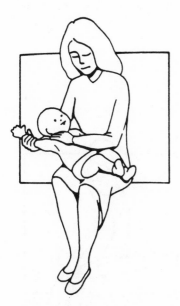

FIG. 1. Draining anterior apical segments.

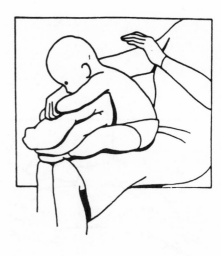

FIG. 2. Draining posterior apical segments.

[a]The material presented here has been reproduced with the kind permission of Dr. Beryl Rosenstein from his excellent booklet, *The Johns Hopkins Hospital Cystic Fibrosis Patient Handbook* (Beryl Rosenstein and Terry S. Langbaum, editors).

189

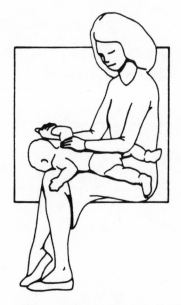

FIG. 3. Draining right posterior segment.

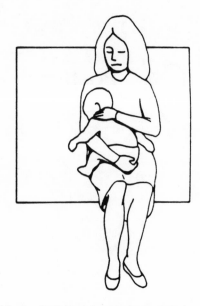

FIG. 4. Draining left posterior segment.

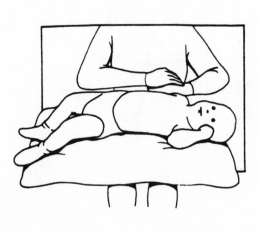

FIG. 5. Draining anterior segments.

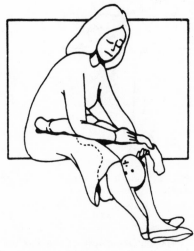

FIG. 6. Draining right middle lobe.

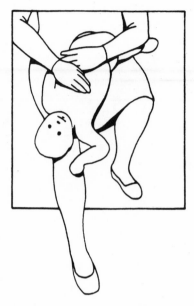

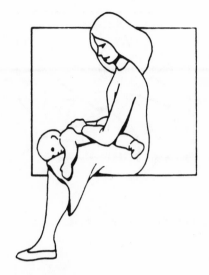

FIG. 8. Draining right and left superior segments.

FIG. 7. Draining left lingula.

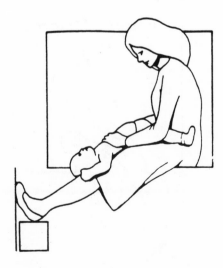

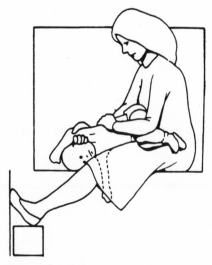

FIG. 9. Draining anterior basal segments.

FIG. 10. Draining left lateral basal segment.

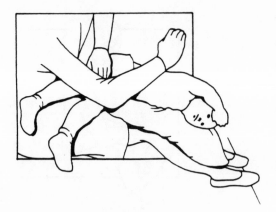

FIG. 11. Draining right lateral basal segment.

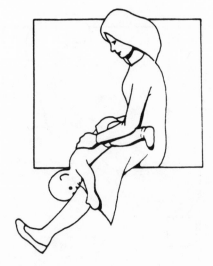

FIG. 12. Draining posterior basal segments.

TODDLERS

The following points will be helpful in performing postural drainage.

• Clap one minute—vibrate five exhalations—vibrate while huffing two to three times, cough, repeat once.
• Each session should last a maximum of 30 to 40 minutes.
• Always do treatment sessions *before* meals.
• Two to three sessions per day are usually recommended.

Other Considerations

Children may become frightened initially when given postural drainage. As this treatment is very important, you should be encouraged not to apologize or sympathize for having to give this form of treatment. Children should understand, to the best of their ability, why the treatment is being done and accept it as part of the daily routine. Children should be encouraged to talk and sing, as this helps them to breathe. Children should not be offered rewards for future treatments. The drainage should be done with as little fuss as possible.

Your child does not need to dislike the time spent in physical therapy. You can make this time a pleasant, quiet opportunity to spend in conversation, or you can provide entertainment by playing records or tapes, or by doing drainage in front of the television.

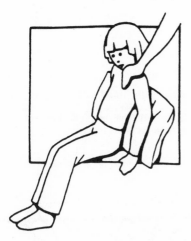

FIG. 13. Upper lobes, apical segments. *Sitting:* Lean back against pillow (30° angle) and clap below collar bone in front with cupped hands.

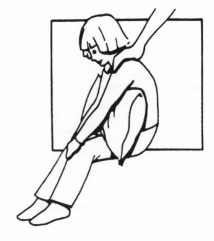

FIG. 14. Upper lobes, posterior segments. *Sitting:* Lean forward onto pillow (30° angle) and clap behind collar bone on the back. The fingers usually go a little over shoulders.

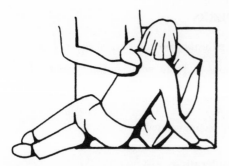

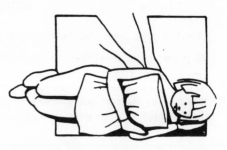

FIG. 15. Left upper lobe. *Bed elevated 45°:* Head up, lying on right side. Place pillow in front, from shoulders to hips, and roll slightly forward onto it. Clap over left shoulder blade.

FIG. 16. Right upper lobe. *Lying on left side:* Place pillow in front, from shoulders to hips, and roll slightly forward onto it. Clap over right shoulder blade.

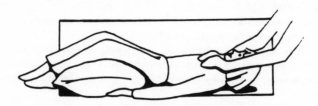

FIG. 17. Upper lobes, anterior segments. *Lying flat on back:* Place pillow under knees and clap just below where you clapped on apical segment.

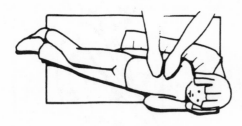

FIG. 18. Right middle lobe. *Lying on left side:* Place pillow behind from shoulders to hips (30° tilt) and roll slightly back onto it (one-quarter turn). Clap over right nipple.

FIG. 19. Left lingula. *Lying on right side:* Place pillow behind, from shoulders to hips, and roll slightly back onto it. Clap over left nipple (30° tilt).

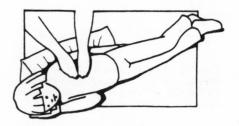

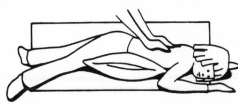

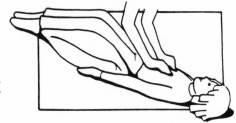

FIG. 20. Lower lobes, superior segments. *Bed flat:* Lying on stomach with pillow under stomach, clap at area of shoulder blades (apex of lower lobes).

FIG. 21. Lower lobes, anterior segments. *Lying on back:* Place pillow under knees and clap on lower ribs (45° tilt).

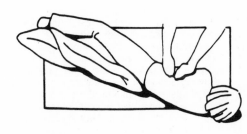

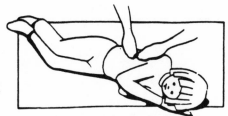

FIG. 22. Lower lobes, left lateral. *Lying on right side:* Knees bent, clap at lower ribs, keeping spine straight (45° tilt).

FIG. 23. Lower lobes, right lateral. *Lying on left side:* Knees bent, clap at lower ribs, keeping spine straight (45° tilt).

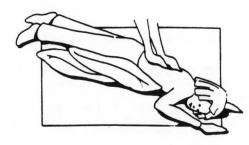

FIG. 24. Lower lobes, posterior segments. *Lying on stomach:* Place pillow under hips and stomach to make spine straight (45° tilt). Clap at lower ribs (stay off spine).

SELF SEGMENTAL BRONCHIAL DRAINAGE

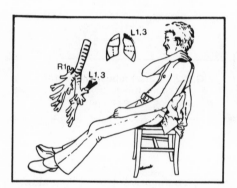

FIG. 25. Sit on a chair and lean backward on a pillow at a 30° angle. Clap with a cupped hand over the area between the clavicle (collarbone) and the top of the scapula (shoulder blade). The area for clapping shown in the diagram is for the *apical*-posterior segment of the left upper lobe, L1,3. The *apical* segment of the right upper lobe, R1, is drained in the same position, with clapping on the right side. **Upper Lobes:** Apical Segments: 1; Apical-Posterior Segment, Left: L1,3; Apical Segment, Right: R3.

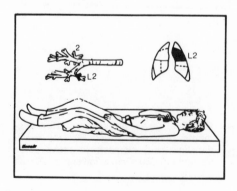

FIG. 26. Lie flat on your back (supine) on a bed or drainage table. Clap between the clavicle (collarbone) and nipple. The area for clapping shown in the diagram is for the *anterior* segment of the left upper lobe, L2. **Upper Lobes:** Anterior Segments: 2.

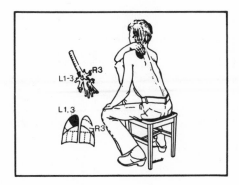

FIG. 27. Sit on a chair leaning forward over a folded pillow at a 30° angle. Clap over the upper back. The area for clapping shown in the diagram is for the apical-*posterior* segment of the left upper lobe, L1-3. The *posterior* segment of the right upper lobe, R3, is drained in the same position with clapping on the right side of the upper back. **Upper Lobes:** Posterior Segments: 3; Posterior Segment, Right: R3; Apical-Posterior Segment, Left: L1-3.

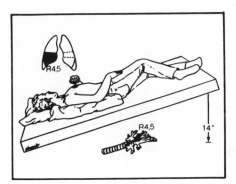

FIG. 28. The foot of the table or bed is elevated 14 inches (about 15°). Lie head down on the left side and rotate 1/4 turn backward. A pillow may be placed behind the back (from shoulder to hip). The knees should be flexed. Clap over the area of the right nipple. Women should use a cupped hand with the heel of the hand under the armpit and the fingers extending forward beneath the breast. The area for clapping of the right *middle lobe,* R4,5, is shown in the diagram. **Right Middle Lobe:** R4,5; Lateral Segment: R4; Medial Segment: R5.

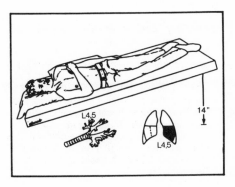

FIG. 29. The *lingular* segment of the left upper lobe, L4,5, is drained by lying in a head-down position on the right side and rotating 1/4 turn backward. Clap over the area of the left nipple. Women should use a cupped hand with the heel of the hand under the armpit and the fingers extending forward beneath the breast. A pillow may be placed behind the back for support. **Lingular Segment, Left Upper Lobe:** L4,5; Superior Segment: L4; Inferior Segment; L5.

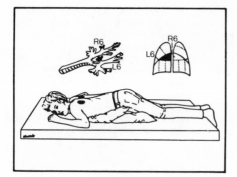

FIG. 30. Lie on your abdomen on a bed or table which is in a flat position with two pillows under your hips. Clap over the middle part of the back at the tip of the scapula (shoulder blade) on either side of the spine. The area for clapping of the *superior* segment of the left lower lobe, L6, is shown in the diagram. The *superior* segment of the right lower lobe, R6, is done in the same position, with clapping on the right side. **Lower Lobes:** Superior Segments: 6.

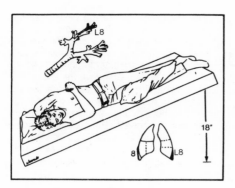

FIG. 31. The foot of the table or bed is elevated 18 inches (about 30°). Lie on your side at a 90° angle in the head-down position with a pillow under your knees. Clap with a cupped hand over the lower ribs just beneath the axilla (armpit). The area for clapping shown is for drainage of the left *anterior basal* segment, L8. To drain the right *anterior basal* segment, R8, lie on your left side in the same position and clap over the right side of the chest. **Lower Lobes:** Anterior Basal Segments: 8.

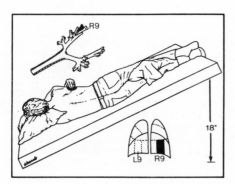

FIG. 32. The foot of the table is elevated 18 inches (approximately 30°). Lie on your abdomen, head down, and rotate 1/4 turn upward from a prone position. Flex your upper leg over a pillow for support. Clap over the lower ribs. The area for clapping shown in the diagram is for the drainage of the right *lateral basal* segment, R9. To drain the left *lateral basal* segment, L9, lie on your right side in the same position and clap over the lower ribs on the left side of the chest. **Lower Lobes:** Lateral Basal Segments: 9.

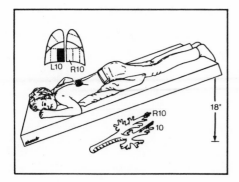

FIG. 33. The foot of the bed or table is elevated 18 inches (about 30°). Lie on your abdomen, head down, with a pillow under your hips. Try to clap over the lower ribs close to the spine. The area for clapping shown in the diagram is for drainage of the *posterior basal* segment of the left lower lobe, L10. For drainage of the *posterior basal* segment of the right lower lobe, lie in the same position and try to clap over the lower ribs on the right side of the chest. This is a difficult area for some individuals to reach and you may want to obtain assistance in clapping in this position. **Lower Lobes:** Posterior Basal Segments: 10.

The History of CF

Some highlights in the History of Cystic Fibrosis are:

1705   A book of folk philosophy states that a salty taste means that a child is bewitched.

1857   *The Almanac of Children's Songs and Games* from Switzerland quotes from Middle Ages:

> "woe is the child who tastes salty from a kiss on the brow, for he is hexed, and soon must die."

1938   Andersen first describes CF, calling it cystic fibrosis of the pancreas.

1946   di Sant'Agnese and Andersen report using antibiotics to treat CF lung infection.

1953   di Sant'Agnese and colleagues describe the sweat abnormality in CF.

1955   First review of use of pancreatic enzymes.

1959   Gibson and Cook describe a safe and accurate way to do sweat testing.

1964   Doershuk, Matthews, and colleagues describe a modern comprehensive treatment program.

1978   First use of enteric-coated pancreatic enzymes.

1981   Description by Knowles and colleagues and Quinton and coworkers of elec-
to   trolyte transport abnormalities.
1983

1986   CF gene localized to chromosome 7.

Modified from Taussig, L. M. *Cystic Fibrosis*, New York: Thieme-Stratton Inc., 1984.

E

CF Care Centers
in the United States

Following is a state-by-state listing of all of the Cystic Fibrosis Care Centers approved by the National Cystic Fibrosis Foundation of the United States, as of 1989. Information about cystic fibrosis organizations in other countries is presented in Appendix F.

ALABAMA

The Children's Hospital
University of Alabama in Birmingham
1600 7th Avenue, South
Birmingham, Alabama 35233
(205) 939–9583
Center Director:
Dana Brasfield, M.D.

University of South Alabama Cystic
Fibrosis Center
USA Children's Speciality Center
Health Services Building, Room 101-D
307 North University Boulevard
Mobile, Alabama 36688
(205) 460–7100
Center Director:
Robert O. Harris III, M.D.

ARIZONA

Cystic Fibrosis Center
Phoenix Children's Hospital
909 East Brill Street
Phoenix, Arizona 85006
(602) 239–5778
Center Director:
Lucy S. Hernried, M.D.

Tucson Cystic Fibrosis Center
St. Luke's Chest Clinic
Arizona Health Sciences Center
1501 North Campbell Avenue
Tucson, Arizona 85724
(602) 626–7450
Center Director:
Richard J. Lemen, M.D.

ARKANSAS

Arkansas Cystic Fibrosis Center
Arkansas Children's Hospital
800 Marshall Street
Little Rock, Arkansas 72202
(501) 370–1018
Center Director:
Karl Karlson, Jr., M.D.

CALIFORNIA

Cystic Fibrosis Center
Miller Children's Hospital Medical
Center
2801 Atlantic Avenue
Long Beach, California 90801
(213) 595–3290
Center Director:
Eliezer Nussbaum, M.D.

Cystic Fibrosis Center
Cedars Sinai Medical Center
8700 Beverly Boulevard
Suite 4430
Los Angeles, California 90048
(213) 855–4421
Center Director:
  Benjamin Kagan, M.D.

Cystic Fibrosis Care, Teaching and
  Resource Center
Children's Hospital of Los Angeles
University of Southern California
  Medical School
4650 Sunset Boulevard
Los Angeles, California 90027
(213) 669–2287
Center Director:
  Chun-I Wang, M.D.

Pediatric Pulmonary Center
Children's Hospital—Oakland
747 52nd Street
Oakland, California 94609
(415) 428–3305
Center Director:
  Nancy C. Lewis, M.D.

Satellite Center:
  Valley Children's Hospital Pediatric
  Pulmonary and Respiratory Care
  3151 North Milbrook
  Fresno, California 93703
  Director
    John Rogers, M.D.

Cystic Fibrosis and Pediatric
  Pulmonary Care, Teaching, and
  Resource Center*
Children's Hospital of Orange County
455 South Main Street
Orange, California 92668
(714) 532–8624
Center Director:
  Ralph W. Rucker, M.D.
Preferred Mailing Address:
  P. O. Box 5700
  Orange, California 92667

Pediatric Pulmonary Disease Center
Children's Hospital at Stanford
520 Sand Hill Road
Palo Alto, California 94304
(415) 853–3377 Ext. 238
Center Director:
  Norman J. Lewiston, M.D.

Cystic Fibrosis and Pediatric
  Respiratory Diseases Center**
University of California at Davis
  School of Medicine
Department of Pediatrics
4301 X Street
Sacramento, California 95817
(916) 453–3189
Center Director:
  Ruth McDonald, M.D.

Brian Wesley Ray CF Center
San Bernardino County Medical
  Center
780 East Gilbert Street
San Bernardino, California 92404
(714) 387–8155 or 3216

San Diego Cystic Fibrosis and
  Pediatric Pulmonary Disease Center
University Hospital
225 West Dickinson Street
San Diego, California 92103
(619) 294–6125
Center Director:
  Ivan R. Harwood, M.D.
  4130 Front Street
  San Diego, California 92103

Kaiser Permanente Medical Care
  Group
900 Kiely Boulevard
Santa Clara, California 95051
(408) 985–4898
Center Director:
  Margaret Delano, M.D.
Cystic Fibrosis Coordinator:
  Gail Farmer, R.D.
**Center includes four locations—call*
  for information.

Cystic Fibrosis Center
University of California at San
   Francisco, Room M687
505 Parnassus Avenue
San Francisco, California 94143
(415) 476–2072
Center Director:
   Brian Davis, M.D.

COLORADO

University of Colorado
Health Science Center
4200 East Ninth Avenue, C220
Denver, Colorado 80262
(303) 394–7518 or 8423
Center Director:
   Frank J. Accurso, M.D.
Satellite Center:
   Billings Clinic
   2825 8th Avenue, North
   Billings, Montana 59101
   (406) 256–2500
   Director:
      Nicholas Wolter, M.D.

CONNECTICUT

Cystic Fibrosis Center
St. Francis Hospital and Medical
   Center
114 Woodland Street
Hartford, Connecticut 06105
(203) 548–4355
Center Director:
   Michelle M. Cloutier, M.D.
   University of Connecticut Health
      Center L-5090
   Farmington, Connecticut 06032

Cystic Fibrosis Center
Yale University School of Medicine
333 Cedar Street
New Haven, Connecticut 06510
(203) 785–2480
Center Director:
   Thomas F. Dolan, Jr., M.D.
   Primary Care Center
   Yale–New Haven Hospital
   20 York Street
   New Haven, Connecticut 06504

DELAWARE

See listing for Satellite Center:
   St. Christopher's Hospital for
   Children
   Philadelphia, Pennsylvania.

WASHINGTON, D.C.

Metropolitan D.C. Cystic Fibrosis
   Center for Care, Training and
   Research
Children's Hospital National Medical
   Center
111 Michigan Avenue, N.W.
Washington, D.C. 20010
(202) 745–2128 or 2129
Center Director:
   Robert J. Fink, M.D.

Georgetown University Cystic
   Fibrosis Center
Georgetown University Medical
   Center
3800 Reservoir Road, N.W. K/C 211
Washington, D.C. 20007
(202) 687–4641
Center Director:
   Lucas L. Kulczycki, M.D.

FLORIDA

Cystic Fibrosis and Pediatric
   Pulmonary Disease Center
University of Florida
Box J-296, Hillis Miller Health Center
Gainesville, Florida 32610
(904) 392–4458
Center Director:
   Sarah E. Chesrown, M.D.

Pediatric Pulmonary and Cystic
   Fibrosis Center
Baptist Medical Center
800 Prudential Drive
Jacksonville, Florida 32207
(904) 390–3788
Center Director:
   Ian Nathanson, M.D.

Cystic Fibrosis Center
Orlando Regional Medical Center
1414 S. Kuhl Avenue
Orlando, Florida 32806
(407) 841–5111, Ext. 6274
Center Director:
   Norman A. Helfrich, Jr., M.D.
   1131 S. Orange Avenue
   Orlando, Florida 32806

University of South Florida
College of Medicine
Department of Pediatrics
Box 15
12901 Bruce B. Downs Boulevard
Tampa, Florida 33612
(813) 974–4214
Center Director:
   James M. Sherman, M.D.

GEORGIA

Emory University
Cystic Fibrosis Center
Department of Pediatrics
2040 Ridgewood Drive, N.E.
Atlanta, Georgia 30322
(404) 727–5728
Center Director:
   Daniel B. Caplan, M.D.

Department of Pediatrics
Section of Pulmonology
Medical College of Georgia
Augusta, Georgia 30912
(404) 721–4723
Acting Center Director:
   Lou Guill, M.D.

Outreach Clinic:
   Ware County Health Department
   604 Riverside Drive
   Waycross, Georgia
   (912) 283–1875

HAWAII

Pediatric Pulmonary and Cystic
   Fibrosis Center
University of Hawaii School of
   Medicine
Kapiolani Women's and Children's
   Medical Center
1319 Punahou Street
Honolulu, Hawaii 96826
(808) 947–8511
Center Director:
   Michael J. Light, M.D.

IDAHO

See listing for Satellite Center:
   University of Utah Medical Center
   Salt Lake City, Utah

ILLINOIS

Cystic Fibrosis Center
Children's Memorial Hospital
Northwestern University
2300 Children's Plaza
Chicago, Illinois 60614
(312) 880–4354
Center Director:
   John D. Lloyd-Still, M.D.

Wyler Children's Hospital
Department of Pediatrics
University of Chicago Hospitals and
   Clinics
Box 133
5841 South Maryland Avenue
Chicago, Illinois 60637
(312) 702–6178
Center Director:
   Lucille A. Lester, M.D.

Pediatric Pulmonary Center
Rush Medical School
Rush-Presbyterian-St. Luke's Medical
Center
1753 West Congress Parkway
Chicago, Illinois 60612
(312) 942–3060
Center Director:
Lewis E. Gibson, M.D.

Outreach Center:
Copley Memorial Hospital
Aurora, Illinois 60505

Cystic Fibrosis Center
Lutheran General Hospital
1775 Dempster Street
Park Ridge, Illinois 60068
(312) 696–7680
Center Director:
Jerome R. Kraut, M.D.

Cystic Fibrosis Center
Saint Francis Medical Center
Specialty Clinics
Hillcrest Medical Plaza
530 N.E. Glen Oak Avenue, 2nd Floor
Peoria, Illinois 61637
(309) 655–4063
Center Director:
Umesh C. Chatrath, M.D.

INDIANA

Cystic Fibrosis and Chronic
Pulmonary Disease Center
Riley Hospital for Children
Indiana University Medical Center
702 Barnhill Drive, Room 293
Indianapolis, Indiana 46223
(317) 274–7208
Center Director:
Howard Eigen, M.D.

Satellite Center:
The Carle Clinic Association
602 W. University Avenue
Urbana, Illinois 61801
Co-Directors:
John A. Moore, M.D.
Terry F. Hatch, M.D.
Outreach Clinic:
Lutheran Hospital
Ft. Wayne, Indiana 46807
Director:
James Pushpom, M.D.

Cystic Fibrosis and Chronic
Pulmonary Disease Clinic
St. Joseph's Medical Center
811 East Madison
South Bend, Indiana 46634
(219) 234–9555
Center Director:
Edward A. Gergesha, M.D.
720 East Cedar
South Bend, Indiana 46617

Cystic Fibrosis & Chronic Pulmonary
Disease Clinic
Elkhart General Hospital
P.O. Box 201
Elkhart, Indiana 46515
(219) 293–7741
Center Director:
Orest Dubynsky, M.D.
1627 E. Bristol Street
Elkhart, Indiana 46514

IOWA

Iowa Methodist Medical Center
Raymond Blank Memorial Hospital
for Children
1200 Pleasant Street
Des Moines, Iowa 50309
(515) 283–6152
Center Director:
Veljko Zivkovich, M.D.
1212 Pleasant Street
Suite 110
Des Moines, Iowa 50309

Cystic Fibrosis Center
Pediatric Allergy and Pulmonary
  Division
Department of Pediatrics
University of Iowa Hospitals and
  Clinics
Iowa City, Iowa 52242
(319) 356–1853
Center Director:
  Miles Weinberger, M.D.

KANSAS

Cystic Fibrosis Care and Teaching
  Center
St. Joseph Medical Center
3600 East Harry
Wichita, Kansas 67218
(316) 689–4707
Center Director:
  Leonard L. Sullivan, M.D.

KENTUCKY

Cystic Fibrosis Center
Department of Pediatrics
Room C 410, C 415
University of Kentucky Medical
  Center
800 Rose Street
Lexington, Kentucky 40536-0843
(606) 233–8023
Center Director:
  Jamshed F. Kanga, M.D.

Louisville Children's Chest Center
University of Louisville
Kosair Children's Hospital
200 E. Chestnut Street
Louisville, Kentucky 40202
(502) 562–8830
Center Director:
  Garrett Adams, M.D., M.P.H.
  Kosair Children's Hospital
  P. O. Box 35070
  Louisville, Kentucky 40232-5070

LOUISIANA

New Orleans Pediatric Pulmonary
  Center
Department of Pediatrics
Tulane University School of Medicine
1430 Tulane Avenue
New Orleans, Louisiana 70112
(504) 588–5601
Center Director:
  Robert C. Beckerman, M.D.

Cystic Fibrosis and Pediatric
  Pulmonary Center
Louisiana State University Medical
  Center
School of Medicine in Shreveport
1501 Kings Highway
P.O. Box 33932
Shreveport, Louisiana 71130-3932
(318) 674–6094
Center Director:
  Bettina C. Hilman, M.D.

MAINE

Cystic Fibrosis Clinical Center
Eastern Maine Medical Center
489 State Street
Bangor, Maine 04401
(207) 947–3711
Co-Center Directors:
  Erlinda A. Polvorosa, M.D.
  John Y. Lambert III, M.D.
  417 State Street
  Bangor, Maine 04401
Outreach Clinic:
  A. R. Gould Memorial Hospital
  Box 151
  Presque Isle, Maine 04769

Central Maine Cystic Fibrosis Center
Central Maine Medical Center
300 Main Street
Lewiston, Maine 04240
(207) 795–2833
Center Director:
  Gilbert R. Grimes, M.D.

Cystic Fibrosis Center
Maine Medical Center
22 Bramhall Street
Portland, Maine 04102
(207) 871–2763
Center Director:
  Nicholas Fowler, M.D.
  Pediatric Center
  229 Vaughn Street
  Portland, Maine 04102

MARYLAND

The Johns Hopkins Hospital
CMSC 149
600 N. Wolfe Street
Baltimore, Maryland 21205
(301) 955–2795
Center Director:
  Beryl J. Rosenstein, M.D.

Cystic Fibrosis Center
National Institute of Diabetes and
  Digestive and Kidney Diseases
National Institutes of Health
Building 10, Room 9D48
Bethesda, Maryland 20892
(301) 496–3434
Center Director:
  Milica S. Chernick, M.D.

MASSACHUSETTS

Cystic Fibrosis Center
Children's Hospital Medical Center
300 Longwood Avenue
Boston, Massachusetts 02115
(617) 735–7881
Center Director:
  Mary Ellen Wohl, M.D.

Cystic Fibrosis Center
Massachusetts General Hospital
ACC 609
15 Parkman Street
Boston, Massachusetts 02114
(617) 726–8707 or 8708
Center Director:
  Allen Lapey, M.D.

Cystic Fibrosis Center
New England Medical Center
  Hospitals, Inc.
Box 343
750 Washington Street
Boston, Massachusetts 02111
(617) 956–5085
Center Director:
  Henry L. Dorkin, M.D.

Baystate Medical Center
Wesson Memorial Unit, 4th Floor
140 High Street
Springfield, Massachusetts 01199
(413) 784–5062
Center Director:
  Robert S. Gerstle, M.D.

MICHIGAN

University of Michigan
Cystic Fibrosis Center
Mott Hospital
F2826, Box 0218
Ann Arbor, Michigan 48109-0010
(313) 764–4123 (Pediatric)
(313) 936–5526 (Adult)
Center Director:
  William F. Howatt, M.D.

Cystic Fibrosis Care, Teaching and
  Resource Center
Children's Hospital of Michigan
Wayne State University Medical
  School
3901 Beaubien Boulevard
Detroit, Michigan 48201
(313) 745–5541
Center Director:
  Robert Wilmott, M.D.
Adult Satellite Network:
  Harper–Grace Hospital
  3990 John R.
  Detroit, Michigan 48201
  (313) 745–8040
  Director:
    Patricia Lynne-Davies, M.D., Ph.D.

Henry Ford Hospital
2799 West Grand Boulevard
Detroit, Michigan 48202
(313) 876–2439
Director:
 Paul A. Kvale, M.D.

Sinai Hospital of Detroit
6767 W. Outer Drive
Detroit, Michigan 48235-2899
Director:
 Alvaro Skupin, M.D.

Satellite Center:
 Mott Children's Health Center
 806 Tuuri Place
 Flint, Michigan 48503
 (313) 767–5750, Ext. 303
 Director:
  Frederick S. Lim, M.D.

Cystic Fibrosis Center
Butterworth Hospital
100 Michigan Street, N.E.
Grand Rapids, Michigan 49503
(616) 774–1712
Center Director:
 Lawrence E. Kurlandsky, M.D.

Greater Lansing Cystic Fibrosis
 Center
Ingham Medical Center
401 West Greenlawn Avenue
Lansing, Michigan 48910
(517) 374–2327
Center Director:
 Richard E. Honicky, M.D.
 B-340 Life Sciences Building
 Michigan State University
 East Lansing, Michigan 48824
Outreach Clinic:
 Clinical Center
 Michigan State University

MINNESOTA

University of Minnesota
Minneapolis, Minnesota 55455
(612) 624–0962
Center Director:
 Warren J. Warwick, M.D.
 Box 184 Mayo Memorial Building
 420 Delaware Street, SE
 Minneapolis, Minnesota 55455
Satellite Center:
 Dakota Medical Center
 1702 S. University Drive
 Fargo, North Dakota 58103
 (701) 280–3373
 Director:
  John G. Wahlstrom, M.D.

MISSISSIPPI

University of Mississippi Medical
 Center
Department of Pediatrics
2500 North State Street
Jackson, Mississippi 39216-4505
(601) 984–5205
Center Director:
 Suzanne T. Miller, M.D.

MISSOURI

Columbia Cystic Fibrosis, Pediatric
 Pulmonary and Gastrointestinal
 Center
University of Missouri Medical Center
Department of Child Health
One Hospital Drive
Columbia, Missouri 65212
(314) 882–6921
Center Director:
 Guilio Barbero, M.D.
Outreach Clinics:
 Medical Gardens
 Suite 107
 2030 South National
 Springfield, Missouri 65802

 Southeast Missouri Hospital
 1701 Lacey Street
 Cape Girardeau, Missouri 63701

The Hannibal Clinic
711 Grand
Hannibal, Missouri 63401

Contact for Outreach Clinics:
Debra A. Morris, R.N., M.S.
(314) 882–6993

The Children's Mercy Hospital
University of Missouri,
  Kansas City School of Medicine
24th and Gillham Road
Kansas City, Missouri 64108
(816) 234–3015
(816) 234–3230 Sweat Test Only
Center Director:
Charles C. Roberts, M.D.

Cystic Fibrosis, Pediatric Pulmonary
  and Pediatric Gastrointestinal
  Center
Cardinal Glennon Memorial Hospital
  for Children
St. Louis University School of
  Medicine
1465 South Grand Boulevard
St. Louis, Missouri 63104
(314) 577–5641
Center Director:
Anthony J. Regent, M.D.
Medical Staff Office
Cardinal Glennon Memorial
  Hospital
1465 South Grand Boulevard
St. Louis, Missouri 63104

St. Louis Children's Hospital
Washington University School of
  Medicine
400 South Kingshighway
Post Office Box 14871
St. Louis, Missouri 63178
(314) 454–6205
Center Director:
Robert J. Rothbaum, M.D.
Satellite Center:
Southern Illinois Medical School
Springfield, Illinois 62708
Director:
Lanie E. Eagleton, M.D.

NEBRASKA

Omaha Center for Cystic Fibrosis and
  Pediatric Pulmonary Diseases
University of Nebraska Hospital
42nd and Dewey Avenue
Omaha, Nebraska 68105
(402) 559–4156
Center Director:
John L. Colombo, M.D.

NEW HAMPSHIRE

New Hampshire Cystic Fibrosis Care
  and Teaching Center
c/o Mary Hitchcock Memorial
  Hospital
2 Maynard Street
Hanover, New Hampshire 03576
(603) 271–4513 or (800) 852–3345 (NH
  only)
Center Director:
William E. Boyle, M.D.
Hitchcock Clinic
2 Maynard Street
Hanover, New Hampshire 03756

NEW JERSEY

University of Medicine and Dentistry
  of New Jersey
New Jersey Medical School
185 South Orange Avenue
Room MSB-F534
Newark, New Jersey 07103-2757
(201) 456–4815
Center Director:
Nelson L. Turcios, M.D.
Satellite Centers:
Cystic Fibrosis Center
Hackensack Medical Center
30 Prospect Avenue
Hackensack, New Jersey 07601
(201) 441–2121
Director:
Lawrence J. Denson, M.D.

Cystic Fibrosis and Chronic
  Pulmonary Disease Center
Monmouth Medical Center
307 Third Avenue
Long Branch, New Jersey 07740
(201) 870–5106
Center Director:
  Robert L. Zanni, M.D.

NEW MEXICO

University of New Mexico
  School of Medicine
Department of Pediatrics
Surge Building
Albuquerque, New Mexico 87131
(505) 277–5551
Center Director:
  Shirley Murphy, M.D.

NEW YORK

Pediatric Pulmonary and Cystic
  Fibrosis Center
Albany Medical College of Union
  University
22 New Scotland Avenue
Albany, New York 12208
(518) 432–1392
Center Director:
  Glenna B. Winnie, M.D.

Long Island College Hospital
340 Henry Street
Brooklyn, New York 11201
(718) 780–1025 or 1026
Center Director:
  Robert Giusti, M.D.

Children's Lung and Cystic Fibrosis
  Center
Children's Hospital of Buffalo
219 Bryant Street
Buffalo, New York 14222
(716) 878–7524

Cystic Fibrosis and Pediatric
  Pulmonary Center
Schneider Children's Hospital of Long
  Island
Jewish Hillside Medical Center
Health Science Center
New Hyde Park, New York 11042
(718) 470–3250
Center Director:
  Jack D. Gorvoy, M.D.

Cystic Fibrosis and Pediatric
  Pulmonary Center
Mount Sinai School of Medicine
Mount Sinai Medical Center
One Gustave L. Levy Place
Fifth Avenue at 100th Street
New York, New York 10029
(212) 650–7788
Center Director:
  Richard J. Bonforte, M.D.
  Director of Pediatrics
  Beth Israel Medical Center
  First Avenue at 16th Street
  New York, New York 10003

Pediatric Pulmonary Center
Babies Hospital and Columbia
  University College of Physicians
  and Surgeons
630 West 168th Street (BHS 101)
New York, New York 10032
(212) 305–5122
Center Director:
  Robert B. Mellins, M.D.

Cystic Fibrosis, Pediatric Pulmonary
  and Gastrointestinal Center
St. Vincent's Hospital and Medical
  Center of New York
36 Seventh Avenue, Suite 509
New York, New York 10011
(212) 790–8895 or 8898
Center Director:
  Carolyn R. Denning, M.D.
Outreach Clinic:
  St. Vincent's Medical Center of
  Richmond
  355 Bard Avenue
  Staten Island, New York 10310

Strong Memorial Hospital
Department of Pediatrics
601 Elmwood Avenue, Box 667
Rochester, New York 14642
(716) 275–5611
Center Director:
John T. McBride, M.D.

Robert C. Schwartz Cystic Fibrosis
Center
State University Hospital
Upstate Medical Center
750 East Adams St.
Syracuse, New York 13210
(315) 473–5834
Center Director:
Phillip T. Swender, M.D.

Cystic Fibrosis Center
Westchester Medical Center
New York Medical College
Valhalla, New York 10595
(914) 347–7570
Center Director:
Armond V. Mascia, M.D.
53 Rose Hill Avenue
Tarrytown, New York 10591

Cystic Fibrosis Center
House of The Good Samaritan
830 Washington Street
Watertown, New York 13601
(315) 785–4072
Center Director:
Ronald G. Perciaccante, M.D.
145 Clinton Street
Watertown, New York 13601

Good Samaritan Hospital (GSH)
1000 Montauk Highway
West Islip, New York 11795
(516) 957–4092
Center Director:
Walter J. O'Connor, M.D.

NORTH CAROLINA

U.N.C. Cystic Fibrosis Center
University of North Carolina
Department of Pediatrics CB7220
509 Burnett-Womack Building
Chapel Hill, North Carolina 27514
(919) 966–1001 (Pediatrics)
(919) 966–1077 (Adults)
Center Director:
Gerald W. Fernald, M.D.
Adult CF Clinic:
Michael Knowles, M.D.
Department of Medicine, CB7020
Division of Pulmonary Medicine
U.N.C. Medical School
724 Clinical Sciences Building
Chapel Hill, North Carolina 27599

Cystic Fibrosis and Pediatric
Pulmonary Center
Duke University Medical Center
P. O. Box 2994
Durham, North Carolina 27710
(919) 684–3364 or
(919) 681–3402
Center Director:
Alexander Spock, M.D.

NORTH DAKOTA

Cystic Fibrosis Center
St. Alexius Medical Center
311 North 9th Street
Bismarck, North Dakota 58502
(701) 224–7500
Center Director:
Margaret E. Morgan, M.D.
Heart and Lung Clinic
Morgan & Associates, M.D.'s, P.C.
311 North 9th Street
Bismarck, North Dakota 58502

OHIO

Pediatric Pulmonary Center
Children's Hospital Medical Center of
Akron
281 Locust Street
Akron, Ohio 44308
(216) 379–8530

Center Director:
Robert T. Stone, M.D.
300 Locust St., Suite 200
Akron, Ohio 44302

The Children's Hospital Medical
Center
Chest-CF Division
Department of Pediatrics
University of Cincinnati, College of
Medicine
Bethesda at Elland Avenue
Cincinnati, Ohio 45229
(513) 559–4511
Center Director:
Frank W. Kellogg, M.D.

Cystic Fibrosis and Pediatric
Pulmonary Institute and Center
Rainbow Babies and Childrens
Hospital
Case Western Reserve University
School of Medicine
2101 Adelbert Road
Cleveland, Ohio 44106
(216) 844–3267
Center Director:
Carl F. Doershuk, M.D.

Columbus Children's Hospital
700 Children's Drive
Columbus, Ohio 43205
(614) 461–6819
Director:
Karen McCoy, M.D.

Pediatric Pulmonary Center
The Children's Medical Center
One Children's Plaza
Dayton, Ohio 45404-1815
(513) 226–8375 or 8376
Center Director:
Martha N. Franz, M.D.

Northwest Ohio Cystic Fibrosis and
Pediatric Pulmonary Center
The Toledo Hospital
2142 North Cove Boulevard
Toledo, Ohio 43606
(419) 471–2207
Center Director:
Pierre A. Vauthy, M.D.

OKLAHOMA

Cystic Fibrosis-Pediatric Pulmonary
Center
Oklahoma Children's Memorial
Hospital
University of Oklahoma
Health Science Center
940 Northeast 13th Street
Oklahoma City, Oklahoma 73126
(405) 271–6390
Center Director:
S. Reyes de La Rocha, M.D.

Tulsa Ambulatory Pediatric Center
2815 South Sheridan Road
Tulsa, Oklahoma 74129
(918) 838–4820
Center Director:
John C. Kramer, M.D.
Utica Square Medical Center
Suite 251
Tulsa, Oklahoma 74114

OREGON

Cystic Fibrosis Care, Teaching and
Research Center
Oregon Health Sciences University
3181 S.W. Sam Jackson Park Road
Portland, Oregon 97201
(503) 279–8503
Center Director:
Michael Wall, M.D.

Outreach Clinic:
Medford CF Clinic
Rogue Valley Hospital
Medford, Oregon 97501

PENNSYLVANIA

Cystic Fibrosis Center
Polyclinic Medical Center
Third and Polyclinic Avenues
Harrisburg, Pennsylvania 17110
(717) 782–4650

Center Director:
James E. Jones, M.D.
Uptown Professional Bldg.
2645 North Third Street
Suite 150
Harrisburg, Pennsylvania 17110

Cystic Fibrosis Center for Care,
Teaching and Research
The Children's Hospital of
Philadelphia
University of Pennsylvania School of
Medicine
34th and Civic Center Boulevard
Philadelphia, Pennsylvania 19104
(215) 596–9582
Center Director:
Thomas F. Scanlin, M.D.
Cystic Fibrosis Center
The Children's Hospital of
Pennsylvania, Room 6125
34th & Civic Center Boulevard
Philadelphia, Pennsylvania 19104

Cystic Fibrosis and Pediatric
Pulmonary Center
Hahnemann University
230 North Broad Street
Philadelphia, Pennsylvania 19102
(215) 448–7766
Center Director:
Douglas S. Holsclaw, Jr., M.D.
Hahnemann University
235 North 15th Street, Room 18123
Philadelphia, Pennsylvania 19102

St. Christopher's Hospital for
Children
Temple University School of Medicine
5th Street and Lehigh Avenue
Philadelphia, Pennsylvania 19133
(215) 427–5183
Center Director:
Daniel V. Schidlow, M.D.
Satellite Centers:
Wilmington Medical Center
501 W. 14th Street (P. O. Box 1668)
Wilmington, Delaware 19899
(302) 428–2661
Director:
Elizabeth M. Craven, M.D.

Geisinger Medical Center
Danville, Pennsylvania 17822
Director:
Stephen Wolf, M.D.
Outreach Clinic:
Mercy Hospital
25 Church Street
Wilkes–Barre, Pennsylvania 18765

Cystic Fibrosis Center
Children's Hospital of Pittsburgh
University of Pittsburgh School of
Medicine
One Children's Place
3705 Fifth Avenue at DeSoto Street
Pittsburgh, Pennsylvania 15213
(412) 692–5630
Center Director:
David M. Orenstein, M.D.

PUERTO RICO

Cystic Fibrosis Care and Teaching
Center
Pediatric Pulmonary Program
Department of Pediatrics
University of Puerto Rico Medical
Sciences Campus
G.P.O. Box 5067
Rio Piedras, Puerto Rico 00936
(809) 763–4966
Center Director:
Pedro M. Mayol, M.D.

RHODE ISLAND

Cystic Fibrosis Center
Rhode Island Hospital
593 Eddy Street
Providence, Rhode Island 02902
(401) 277–5685
Center Director:
Mary Ann Passero, M.D.

SOUTH CAROLINA

Cystic Fibrosis Center
Medical University of South Carolina
171 Ashley Avenue
Charleston, South Carolina 29425
(803) 792–3561
Center Director:
  Margaret Q. Jenkins, M.D.

SOUTH DAKOTA

South Dakota Cystic Fibrosis Center
Sioux Valley Hospital
1100 South Euclid Avenue
Sioux Falls, South Dakota 57117-5039
(605) 333–7189
Center Director:
  Rodney R. Parry, M.D.

TENNESSEE

Memphis Cystic Fibrosis Center
Le Bonheur Children's Medical Center
University of Tennessee Center for the
  Health Sciences
One Children's Plaza
Memphis, Tennessee 38103
(901) 522–3302
Center Director:
  Philip George, M.D.
  Section of Respiratory Diseases
  Le Bonheur Children's Medical
    Center
  848 Adams Avenue
  Memphis, Tennessee 38103

Vanderbilt University Medical Center
2948 The Vanderbilt Center
Nashville, Tennessee 37232
(615) 322–6134
Center Director:
  Preston W. Campbell, III, M.D.

TEXAS

Cystic Fibrosis Care, Teaching and
  Research Center
Children's Medical Center
1935 Motor Street, Room 316
Dallas, Texas 75235
(214) 920–2361 or 2362
Center Director:
  Robert I. Kramer, M.D.
Satellite Center:
  Permian Basin Allergy Center
  606 North Kent Street
  Midland, Texas 79701
Director:
  John D. Bray, M.D.

Cystic Fibrosis Center
Cook-Ft. Worth Children's Medical
  Center
801 Seventh Avenue
Fort Worth, Texas 76104
(817) 885–4000, Ext. 116
Co-Directors:
  James C. Cunningham, M.D.
  Nancy Dambro, M.D.

Cystic Fibrosis Center
Pulmonary Section
Department of Pediatrics
Baylor College of Medicine
One Baylor Plaza
Houston, Texas 77030
(713) 665–3312
Center Director:
  Dan K. Seilheimer, M.D.
  2201 W. Holcombe
  Suite 310
  Houston, Texas 77030

Satellite Center:
  The University of Texas Health
    Center at Tyler
  P. O. Box 2003
  Tyler, Texas 75710
  (214) 877–7220
  Co-Directors:
    Michael Green, M.D.
    Philip Black, M.D.

Outreach Clinic:
Cystic Fibrosis and Related
  Respiratory Disease Program
Seton Medical Center
1201 West 38th Street
Austin, Texas 78705
(512) 459–2121
Director:
  Allan L. Frank, M.D.

Cystic Fibrosis-Chronic Lung Disease
  Center
The Children's Hospital
519 W. Houston Street
P. O. Box 7330, Station A
San Antonio, Texas 78207
(512) 228–2058 or
(512) 228–2201
Center Director:
  Ricardo Pinero, M.D.
  343 West Houston St. #902
  San Antonio, Texas 78205

UTAH

Intermountain Cystic Fibrosis Center
Department of Pediatrics
University of Utah Medical Center
50 North Medical Drive
Salt Lake City, Utah 84132
(801) 581–8227
Acting Center Director:
  Dennis Nielson, M.D.

Satellite Centers:
  Mercy Medical Center
  1512 12th Avenue Road
  Nampa, Idaho 83651
  (208) 467–1171, Ext. 163
  Director:
    Eugene M. Brown, M.D.
    215 East Hawaii
    Nampa, Idaho 83651

  Pediatric Intensive Care & Chest
    Consultants, Chtd.
  2040 W. Charleston Blvd., Suite 401
  Las Vegas, Nevada 89102
  (702) 386–9008
  Co-Directors:
    John R. Carlile, M.D.
    Vincent P. McCarthy, M.D.

VERMONT

Cystic Fibrosis and Pediatric
  Pulmonary Center
Medical Center Hospital of Vermont
University of Vermont
One Kennedy Drive
South Burlington, Vermont 05401
(802) 862–5529
Center Director:
  Donald R. Swartz, M.D.

VIRGINIA

Cystic Fibrosis Care, Teaching and
  Research Center
University of Virginia
School of Medicine
Charlottesville, Virginia 22908
(804) 924–2613
Center Director:
  Robert F. Selden, Jr., M.D.
  University of Virginia Medical
    Center
  Department of Pediatrics
  P. O. Box 501
  Charlottesville, Virginia 22908

Eastern Virginia Medical School
Children's Hospital of the King's
  Daughters
800 West Olney Road, Room 204
Norfolk, Virginia 23507
(804) 628–7238
Center Director:
  Thomas Rubio, M.D.

Cystic Fibrosis Program
Medical College of Virginia
Box 271, MCV Station
Richmond, Virginia 23298
(804) 786–9445
Center Director:
  David A. Draper, M.D.

WASHINGTON

Pulmonary Disease and Cystic
Fibrosis Center
Children's Orthopedic Hospital and
Medical Center
P.O. Box C5371
Seattle, Washington 98105
(206) 526–2024
Center Director:
Bonnie W. Ramsey, M.D.
Satellite Center:
Mary Bridge Children's Health
Center
1811 South "K" Street
Tacoma, Washington 98405
(206) 383–2903
Co-Directors:
Lawrence A. Larson, D.O.
Ross S. Kendall, M.D.

WEST VIRGINIA

Cystic Fibrosis Center for Care,
Teaching and Research
West Virginia University Medical
Center
Morgantown, West Virginia 26506
(304) 293–4452
Center Co-Directors:
Henry L. Abrons, M.D.
Pulmonary Disease Section
Beverly T. Ellington, M.D.
Department of Pediatrics

WISCONSIN

University of Wisconsin
Cystic Fibrosis/Pediatric Pulmonary
Center
Clinical Sciences Center - H4/434
600 Highland Avenue
Madison, Wisconsin 53792
(608) 263–8555
Center Director:
Elaine Mischler, M.D.

Children's Hospital of Wisconsin
Medical College of Wisconsin
1700 West Wisconsin Avenue
Milwaukee, Wisconsin 53233
(414) 931–1010
Center Director:
W. Theodore Bruns, M.D.

CF Organizations Worldwide

ARGENTINA

Dr. O. H. Pivetta, President
Cystic Fibrosis Association of
  Argentina
Beruti 2857 - 40. Piso "16"
1425 Buenos Aires, Argentina

AUSTRALIA

Mr. Eric Ryan, National Secretary
Australian Cystic Fibrosis
  Foundation, Inc.
P.O. Box 225
Paddington, Queensland 4064
Australia

AUSTRIA

Friedrich Komarek, President
Cystic Fibrosis Association
Heilisenkreuzerstr 29A
A 2384 Breitenfurt, Austria

BELGIUM

Mr. Andre George, Secretary General
Association Belge de Lutte Contre la
  Mucoviscidose
Place Georges Brugmann 29
1060 Brussels, Belgium

BRAZIL

Dr. Ludma Trotta Dallalana
Assoc. Brazilara de Assistencia a
  Mucoviscidose
Av. Rui Barbosa
716 Botafogo
Rio de Janeiro, Brazil

CANADA

Mrs. Cathleen Morrison, Executive
  Director
Canadian Cystic Fibrosis Foundation
586 Eglinton Avenue East, Suite 204
Toronto, Ontario M4P 1P2, Canada

CHILE

Patricio Lira Venegas
Corporation Para La Fibrosis Quistica
  del Pancreas
La Canada 6506 (i)
La Reina, Santiago, Chile

CUBA

Dr. Manuel Rojo Concepcion,
  President
Comision Cubana de Fibrosis Quistica
Servicio de Enfermedades Respr.
Hospital Pediatrico Pedro Borres
F entre 27 Y 29
Vedade Habana 4
La Habana, Cuba

CZECHOSLOVAKIA

Dr. V. Vavrova
Cystic Fibrosis Association
Inst. Evolutionis Infantum
 Investigandae
15112 Prague 5-Motol
V Uvalu 84, Czechoslovakia

DENMARK

Mrs. Hanne Wendel Tyokjaer
Landsforeningen Til Bekaempelse af
 Cystisk Fibrose
Hyrdebakken 246
DK-8800 Viborg, Denmark

EGYPT

Dr. Ekram Abdel-Salam
111 Abdel Aziz Suaoud Str.
Manial, Cairo, Egypt

FEDERAL REPUBLIC OF GERMANY

Mr. Wolfgang Hutzler
Deutsche Gesellschaft zur
 Bekampfung der Mucoviscidose e.v.
 Erlangen
Hainstrasse 8, Postfach 1810
8500 Nürnberg, Federal Republic of
 Germany

FRANCE

Mr. Rene Barau, Administrator
Association Francaise de Lutte Contre
 la Mucoviscidose
66 Boulevard St. Michel
75 Paris 6e, France

GERMAN DEMOCRATIC REPUBLIC

Professor H. Dietzsch
Arbeitsgruppe zur Bekampfung der
 Mucoviscidose
Fetcherstrasse 74
8019 Dresden, German Democratic
 Republic

GREECE

Hellenic Cystic Fibrosis Association
Ag. Sikelianou 8
N. Psychico 15452
Athens, Greece

ICELAND

Dr. H. Bergsteinsson
Icelandic Cystic Fibrosis Group
Barnaspitali Hringsins
Landspitalinn u/Baronsstig
Reykjavik–Postholf 101, Iceland

IRELAND

Mr. Ken French, Honorary Secretary
Cystic Fibrosis Association of Ireland
24 Lower Rathmines Road
Dublin 6, Ireland

ISRAEL

Dr. Nathan Durst
Cystic Fibrosis Foundation of Israel
Benjaminstr. 5, P.O. Box 31171
Tel Aviv 61311, Israel

ITALY

Diego Bortolusso, Secretary
Assoc. Italiana per la Contro la
 Fibrosi Cistica
Via Seminario n. 10
30026 Portogruaro
Venezia, Italy

JORDAN

Cystic Fibrosis Jordan
University of Jordan
P.O. Box 13350
Amman, Jordan

MEXICO

Mr. Antonio Gutierrez Cortina,
    President
Assoc. Mexicana de Fibrosis Quistica
Av. Revolucion 1389
01040 Mexico D.F.

THE NETHERLANDS

Mr. H. J. van Lier
Nederlandse Cystic Fibrosis Stichting
c/o Amro Bank, P.O. Box 2059
3500 Utrecht, The Netherlands

NEW ZEALAND

Mr. C. W. McDonald, National
    Secretary
Cystic Fibrosis Association of New
    Zealand
P.O. Box 1755
Wellington, New Zealand

NORWAY

Dr. Per Espeli
Norwegian Cystic Fibrosis
    Association
c/o Norges Handikapforbund
Nils Hansensvei 2
Oslo 6, Norway

POLAND

Professor Krystyna Boskova
Polish Cystic Fibrosis Association
National Institute of Mother and Child
U1 Kasprzaka, 17
Warsaw, Poland

SOUTH AFRICA

Mrs. M. E. Kay
Southern Africa Cystic Fibrosis
    Association
Addington Hospital, Durban
Natal, South Africa

SPAIN

Dr. Jeronimo Pujol, President
Asociacion Espanola Contra la
    Fibrosis Quistica
Avda. S. Antonio M. Claret 167
Barcelona 25, Spain

SWEDEN

Miss Birgitta Carlson
Riskforeningen for Cystisk Fibros
Box 3049
750 03 Uppsala, Sweden

SWITZERLAND

Mr. H. Muller, Secretary
Swiss Cystic Fibrosis Association
Bellevuestrasse 166, P.O. Box 24
CH-3028 Spiegel/BE, Switzerland

TURKEY

Dr. Omar Ozalp
Department of Pediatrics
University of Hacettepe
Ankara, Turkey

UNITED KINGDOM

Mrs. Barbara Bentley
Cystic Fibrosis Research Trust
5 Blyth Road, Bromley
Kent BR1 3BS, UK.

Association of CF Adults (UK)
288 New Road, Ferndown,
Dorset BH22 8EP, UK

UNITED STATES

Robert K. Dresing, President
Cystic Fibrosis Foundation
6931 Arlington Road
Bethesda, Maryland 20814

URUGUAY

Dr. Carlos Boccoleri
Cystic Fibrosis Association of
  Uruguay
Br. Artigas 1465 esq. Palmer
Montevideo, Uruguay

YUGOSLAVIA

Dr. Streten Sicevic
Cystic Fibrosis Association of
  Yugoslavia
Mother and Child Institute of Serbia
8, Radoja Dakica Street
11071 New Belgrade, Yugoslavia

Associate Members of the ICF(M)A[1]

FINLAND

Mr. Ilpo Vikkumaa
Cystic Fibrosis Association of Finland
Keuhkovammaliitto
Pohjoinen Hesperiankatu 15 A
00260 Helsinki 26, Finland

HUNGARY

Dr. Kalman Gyurkovits
N.W.G. for Cystic Fibrosis
Medical University School of Szeged
Koranyi Fasor 18, H-6701
Szeged, P.O. Box 471, Hungary

INDIA

Bhulabhai D. Patel, M.D.
82-B Embassy Apartments
46 Nepean Sea Road
Bombay 36, India

PORTUGAL

Dr. A. Valido
Rua Manuel Faria de Sousa No 16
Santo Amaro de Oeiras
2780 Oeiras, Portugal

USSR

Professor Sergei V. Rachinsky, M.D.
Head, Dept. of Pulmonology
Institute of Paediatrics
Academy of Medical Sciences of the
  USSR
V-292 Lomonosovsky PR 2
Moscow, USSR

Dr. Vladimir K. Tatochenko
Institute of Paediatrics
Academy of Medical Sciences of the
  USSR
V-292 Lomonosovsky PR 2
Moscow, USSR

---

[1]ICF(M)A, International Cystic Fibrosis (Mucoviscidosis) Association

G / Bibliography

SUGGESTED READING

General

Lloyd-Still JD. *Textbook of Cystic Fibrosis*. John Wright PSG Inc., Boston, 1983.
A comprehensive text on cystic fibrosis; an excellent resource.

Taussig LM. *Cystic Fibrosis*. Thieme-Stratton Inc., New York, 1984.
Also a superb comprehensive text.

Davis PB, ed. *Cystic Fibrosis*. Seminars in Respiratory Medicine, 1985; 6(4) (April 1985).
The entire issue is devoted to cystic fibrosis, with individual articles by nationally recognized authorities.

Boat TF. Cystic Fibrosis. In: Murray JF, Nadel JA, eds. *Textbook of Respiratory Medicine*. W.B. Saunders Co., Philadelphia, 1988; 1126–1152.
Superb overview of the field, clearly written, with 207 references.

Scanlin TF. Cystic Fibrosis. In: Fishman AP, ed. *Pulmonary Diseases and Disorders,* 2nd ed. McGraw-Hill Book Company, New York, 1988; 1273–1294.
Another comprehensive overview of the field.

Of Historical Interest

Andersen DH. Cystic fibrosis of the pancreas and its relation to celiac disease; a clinical and pathologic study. *Am J Dis Child* 1938;356:344–395.
The earliest description of cystic fibrosis as a single entity.

di Sant'Agnese PA, Darling RC, Perera GA, Shea E. Abnormal electrolyte composition of sweat in cystic fibrosis of the pancreas. Clinical significance and relationship of the disease. *Pediatrics* 1953;12:549–563.
Original description of the high salt content in CF sweat.

Doershuk CF, Matthews LW, Tucker AS, et al. A five year clinical evaluation of a therapeutic program for patients with cystic fibrosis. *J Pediatr* 1964;65:677ff.
The first paper to show the benefit of a comprehensive treatment program for patients with CF.

Gibson LE, Cooke, RE. A test for concentration of electrolytes in sweat in cystic fibrosis of the pancreas utilizing pilocarpine by iontophoresis. *Pediatrics* 1959;23:545–549.
Landmark report detailing a laboratory method for collection and analysis of CF sweat.

Knowles M, Gatzy J, Boucher R. Increased bioelectric potential difference across respiratory epithelia in cystic fibrosis. *N Engl J Med* 1981;305:1489–1495.
The first of the papers to elucidate the problem with electrolyte transport across mucous membranes in CF.

Quinton PM, Bijman J. Higher bioelectric potentials due to decreased chloride absorption in the sweat glands of patients with cystic fibrosis. *N Engl J Med* 1983;308:1185–1189.
Initial publication demonstrating that the problem in nose and respiratory tree also existed in sweat glands, and that it was primarily a problem with chloride not being able to pass through mucous membranes.

Subject Index